NATURAL PREGNANCY

THE AUTHORS

Lee Rodwell is a leading freelance journalist who specializes in health issues, lifestyle, and family matters. Now Health Editor of the top-selling UK weekly women's magazine, *Take A Break*, she has written extensively for a broad cross-section of Britain's national newspaper and magazine market. She has written numerous articles about pregnancy and childbirth and has contributed features to *Parents* and *Mother and Baby* magazines. Her work regularly appears in a wide range of publications. She is a member of the Guild of Health Writers and the author of six books. Married to a newspaper design consultant, she has sailed through her pregnancies with the help of yoga and herbal tea, had two quick, natural births, and has two healthy school-age children.

Andrea Kon has worked as a leading features writer and journalist for most UK national newspapers and magazines. She specializes in health, complementary medicine, diet, and human interest issues. For several years, whilst on the staff of *TV Times*, she edited Dr Miriam Stoppard's column, and has worked closely with Kathryn Marsden who formulated the Food Combining Diet. Andrea has written widely on issues concerning the health and welfare of mothers-to-be and relationships between parents and children. She actively promotes homeopathy, aromatherapy, and relaxation techniques in pregnancy as a positive avenue to easy childbirth. Andrea, who is widowed, has two adult daughters.

The Institute for Complementary Medicine

The Institute for Complementary Medicine (ICM) was founded in Britain in 1982. It is a charitable organization whose aim is to encourage the development of all forms of complementary medicine, including research, education, and standards of clinical practice, and to provide factual information to the Media and the public. With over 370 affiliated organizations, the ICM sees complementary medicine as a separate and independent source of health care, yet it always encourages a correct relationship with the medical profession to ensure each case receives the most appropriate treatment available.

COMPLEMENTARY HEALTH

NATURAL
PREGNANCY

LEE RODWELL & ANDREA KON

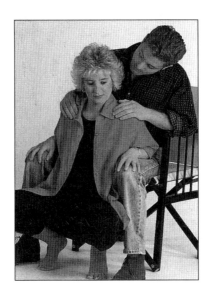

SMITHMARK

A Salamander Book

© Salamander Books Ltd., 1997.
129-137 York Way,
London N7 9LG,
United Kingdom.

This edition published in 1997 by SMITHMARK Publishers,
a division of U.S. Media Holdings, Inc.,
16 East 32nd Street,
New York, NY 10016.

9 8 7 6 5 4 3 2 1

SMITHMARK books are available for bulk purchase for sales promotion and premium use. For details write or call the manager of special sales, SMITHMARK Publishers,
16 East 32nd Street,
New York,
NY 10016; (212) 532–6600

ISBN 0–7651–9957–2

This book was created by SP Creative Design for Salamander Books Ltd.
Editor: Heather Thomas
Designer: Al Rockall
Production: Rolando Ugolini
Illustration reproduction: Emirates Printing Press, Dubai
Printed in Spain

Photography:
Studio photography by Bruce Head
Bubbles: pages 57, 58, 71, 73, 80, 81, 83, 84, 85, 93, 94, 95, 101
The Image Bank: pages 7, 9
Mark Shearman: pages 24, 27
Illustrations on pages 104–107 by A. Milne

IMPORTANT

CONTENTS

PREPARING FOR PREGNANCY   6

GOOD FOOD NATURALLY   16

GET FIT FOR PREGNANCY   24

STAY HEALTHY NATURALLY   44

GET FIT FOR LABOR   56

NATURAL BIRTH   70

COMPLEMENTARY MEDICINE   94

PROGRESS IN PREGNANCY   102

USEFUL ADDRESSES   108

INDEX   111

CHAPTER ONE

PREPARING FOR PREGNANCY

Planning for a family means much more than deciding when to stop using contraception. Ideally, if you are thinking of having a baby, you and your partner should allow yourselves at least six months, if not a year, to ensure that you are both as healthy as possible before you conceive. This gives you time to check your diet and lifestyles and make any necessary changes that could give your child the optimum start in life.

Of course, many bouncing babies are born to mothers who had no idea they were pregnant until they missed a period or two. And there will always be some babies born with unavoidable problems, no matter how carefully their parents prepared and planned. Even so, it makes sense to do all you can to increase your chances of having a trouble-free pregnancy and giving birth to a healthy baby.

HEALTH CHECKS

You can start by going to see your doctor. Even if he cannot give you the proper preconception care and advice you are seeking, he should be able to tell you what care is available.

■ Both you and your partner should be given a physical examination, and checked to ensure that neither of you is suffering from a sexually transmitted disease, including the HIV virus. Depending on when you had your last test, you may be given a cervical smear. You may be screened for breast cancer and given treatment, if necessary, for thrush or candida.

■ You should be given a blood test to see whether you have had rubella (German measles) if you have not been vaccinated against it. Rubella is a very infectious illness which can be so mild that it may pass unnoticed. However, if you catch it in the first three months of pregnancy, it can damage the developing baby. If you need vaccinating against rubella it is important to use a contraceptive and wait for three months before trying to conceive, as a live vaccine is used which could harm a growing fetus.

■ If your own doctor does not offer preconception care, he may refer you to another doctor or clinic where you and your partner can be advised.

HOMEOPATHY

Homeopathy is based on the "like-cures-like" principle. It works by using tiny amounts of natural substances which, if taken in larger doses, would cause

Opposite: both you and your partner can start preparing for pregnancy before the baby is conceived. Start by going to your doctor for a health check.

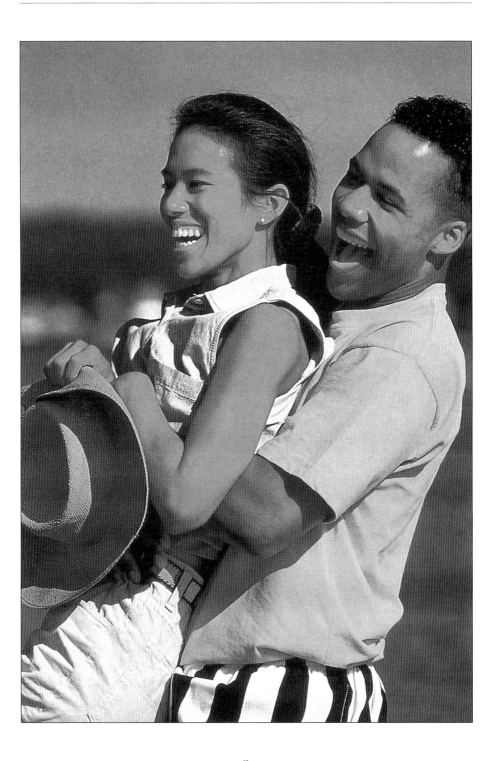

symptoms of the problem from which the patient is suffering.

A visit to a registered homeopath before conception could identify any familial weaknesses that affect your health. The aim of the treatment would be to get your body back in balance, minimizing any susceptibilities. Every individual's personality, emotional state and physical symptoms are matched to a specific remedy. For advice on how to find a registered homeopath, see page 108.

COUNSELING

If you decide to see a counselor for advice, you will almost certainly be asked about your smoking and drinking habits, your use of medication and other drugs, what you eat and how much you weigh, how prone you are to tiredness and stress, and what kind of contraception you have been using.

WHAT TO AVOID

■ SMOKING

This can reduce your chances of getting pregnant: it may reduce a woman's fertility and increase the risk of early miscarriage, whereas men who smoke heavily may have reduced testosterone levels and sperm counts.

If either of you smoke, now is the time to quit. You may need help and support if you are to be successful in doing this. Ask your doctor for advice.

■ ALCOHOL, DRUGS AND MEDICINES

It may also be a good idea to limit your alcohol intake. Try to avoid all drugs or

> ## PRECONCEPTUAL ORGANIZATIONS
>
> These exist in many countries and can be very helpful in advising you on the many aspects of preconceptual care. These organizations are usually set up by parents, doctors, and nutritionists. You and your partner could both pay for a total health analysis at one of their clinics.

medicines, including so-called recreational drugs, such as marijuana, ecstasy and cocaine. Marijuana, for instance, can damage your genetic make-up, while cocaine can affect the sperm mobility.

Of course, if you are taking prescribed drugs for a medical condition you must seek your doctor's advice before you stop or reduce them.

You may want to consider alternative forms of treatment, such as herbal medicine and homeopathic remedies. Although most of these are harmless, it is best to seek qualified advice rather than trying to treat yourself. Yoga, relaxation, reflexology, acupuncture, or hypnotherapy may be preferable to taking pills or potions (see page 108 for contact addresses).

Opposite: once you have made the decision to start a family, you should both try to eat a healthy diet, exercise regularly, limit your alcohol intake, and quit smoking if possible.

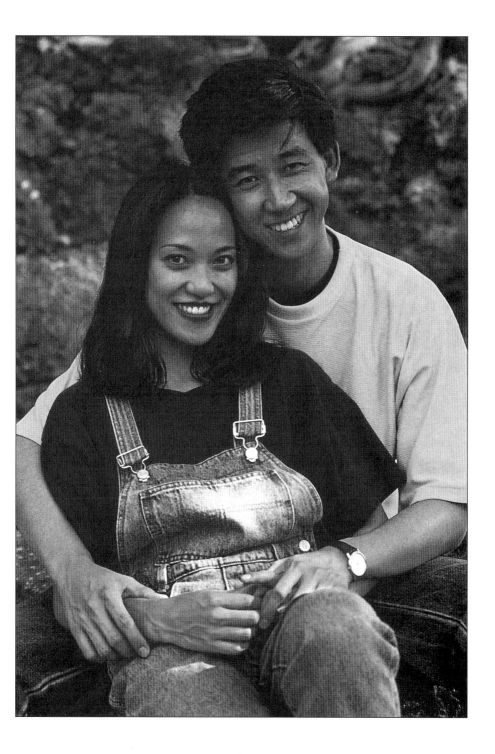

FOOD AND WEIGHT

If you are underweight you may become temporarily infertile and unable to conceive unless you put on a few pounds. If you do fall pregnant, you are more likely to have a smaller baby than a woman of normal weight. However, if you are grossly overweight, you may experience menstrual difficulties and problems during pregnancy.

Your partner's weight can make a difference, too. If he is very fat his fertility may be affected and his sperm count may be lowered. This is why it makes sense to adjust your eating habits, if necessary, well before you start trying for a baby.

The benefits of a natural, pesticide-free diet apply to everyone. Healthy eating should put the emphasis on fresh fruit and vegetables; starchy foods such as bread, potatoes, rice, pasta and breakfast cereals (wholemeal or whole-grain, where possible); lean meat and oily fish; and low-fat dairy products.

Once you start thinking about having a baby, it is worth trying to eat sensibly. You could cut down on processed foods, high-fat foods and foods that contain large amounts of sugar, additives, and colorings. You might prefer to buy organic produce. In any case, you should make sure that you wash all fruit, salads and vegetables thoroughly and avoid raw egg yolks and, if possible, raw or under-cooked meat. When cooking vegetables, try to steam rather than boil them, and remember that over-cooking destroys vitamins.

DRINK

Try to watch what you drink. Apart from cutting down on alcohol, watch your intake of drinks containing caffeine—tea and colas as well as coffee. Instead, drink plenty of water. Your tap water may be contaminated with lead or copper from old piping, so you may prefer to buy bottled carbonated or still water, or to use a filter. Avoid unpasteurized milk, too.

VITAMIN AND MINERAL SUPPLEMENTS AND FOLIC ACID

If you are eating healthily, as suggested above, you will both probably be getting the vitamins and minerals you need from your everyday meals. However, if you are a vegetarian or on a restricted diet for other reasons, you may need to take supplements. Ask your doctor about this.

■ **Folic acid:** this is the one vitamin you should take before you start trying to get pregnant. Adequate intake of folic acid lessens the risk of your having a baby with a central nervous system disorder. You need a 0.4 milligrams tablet every day, and you could continue taking the supplement until you are 12 weeks pregnant. It's also worth knowing that yeast extract and dark green vegetables are rich in folic acid, and that it is added to some foods.

■ **Zinc:** this mineral is found in oily fish, oysters, meat, wheatgerm, brewer's yeast, nuts, pumpkin seeds, onions, peas, and beans. It is an essential nutrient for the manufacture of the genetic material of cells.

■ **Calcium and magnesium:** these are essential for the formation and maintenance of strong bones and healthy teeth. The best dietary sources of magnesium are green, leafy vegetables. Calcium is found in milk and dairy products, sardines, dark green leafy vegetables, dried beans, and nuts. If you can't tolerate milk products, you may wish to consult your doctor about taking a supplement.

MEN SHOULD MAKE SURE THEY EAT PLENTY OF:

■ Food containing vitamin C: fresh fruit, particularly citrus fruit, strawberries, tomatoes, and green vegetables. These foods promote the motility of the sperm.

WOMEN SHOULD MAKE SURE THEY EAT PLENTY OF:

■ Food containing vitamin B, particularly B6: meat, oily fish, brewer's yeast, whole grains, wheatgerm, bananas, avocados, potatoes, and eggs. B6 (pyridoxine) helps the body produce antibodies to fight disease. B1 (thiamine) is needed for fertility. B2 (riboflavin) is essential at the time of conception for normal growth and development of the embryo. B5 (pantothenic acid) is essential for the healthy functioning of the reproductive systems of the body.

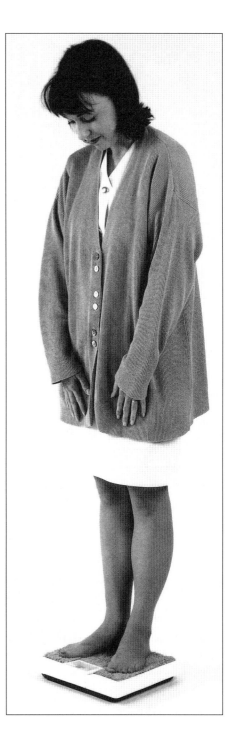

STRESS AND HOW TO CONQUER IT

There is evidence to suggest that stress can affect the health of both men and women. It can affect a man's sperm count, and much otherwise inexplicable infertility may be stress-related.

No matter how hard you try, you won't be able to avoid stress altogether (indeed, experts believe that a certain amount of stress is actually good for us). But you do need to find ways of avoiding overload.

RELAXATION AND MEDITATION

Relaxation is something you can teach yourself. One technique for getting rid of the tensions in your body is discussed in more detail on page 29. Meditation is a way of relaxing the mind. One of the simplest meditation techniques is to find a quiet warm place where you won't be interrupted. Settle yourself comfortably, close your eyes and choose an image to think about. It may be waves breaking on a beach or flowers in a garden. Or you might choose a sound, which you say to yourself every time you breathe out. If other thoughts intrude, just acknowledge them and let them pass. Then bring your mind back to whatever you are focusing on. At first you may be able to carry on like this for only a few minutes, but gradually you should manage to build up to 20 minutes of meditation at a time.

AROMATHERAPY

Massage is another good way of relaxing. Aromatherapy combines massage with the use of essential oils. The healing properties of the plants can be smelled as they are breathed in through your nose and mouth. They are absorbed into your body through your skin.

You can arrange to see a qualified aromatherapist (see page 108) or you can ask your partner to massage you. You can even massage yourself. Work with long, sweeping movements. The beneficial effects of aromatherapy are not confined to massage. Warm baths, scented with essential oil, taken just before bedtime can soak away the troubles of the day.

■ **A few words of warning:** if you think you might already be pregnant, seek advice. Some oils—such as Geranium or Neroli—

Below and opposite: aromatherapy can soothe away stress by combining massage and the use of essential oils which are absorbed through the skin.

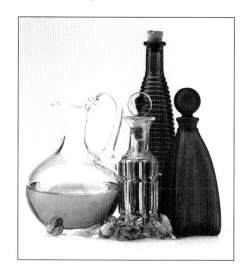

should be avoided in pregnancy. Never use essential oils direct on to the skin. Never use them if you have a migraine, or if your skin is inflamed, broken or infected, or over varicose veins.

ESSENTIAL OILS THAT PROMOTE GOOD HEALTH AND AID CONCEPTION

■ **Geranium:** eases premenstrual tension,

aids fertility, balances the body's hormones, relieves stress and tension, improves circulation.

■ **Clary, Jasmine, Neroli, Patchouli, Rose, Sandalwood, Ylang Ylang:** have aphrodisiac qualities, and help in the treatment of impotence or frigidity.

■ **Frankincense, Lavender, Neroli, Rose, Ylang Ylang:** soothing and calming.

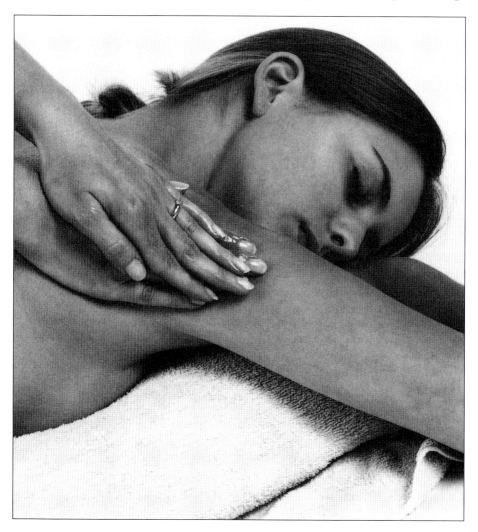

ENVIRONMENTAL HAZARDS

For most of us it is impossible to avoid the exhaust fumes, smoke, and other pollutants that pervade so many towns and cities. However, knowing where the hidden hazards lurk is the first step towards changing some aspects of your everyday life which may affect your health and your chances of conceiving and carrying a healthy baby.

■ **Carbon monoxide:** those at risk include anyone working with or near gas and diesel engines and gas heaters. Small amounts are found in laser printers and photocopiers. This gas is also a significant by-product of tobacco smoking.

■ **Carbon disulphide:** used in the manufacture of plastics and other manufacturing processes. Can cause sexual dysfunction in both sexes.

■ **Formaldehyde:** those at risk include people working in hospitals, particularly operating theaters, furniture and construction workers, and those involved in manufacturing plastics, paints, foams, and resins. Can cause sterility in women.

■ **Metals:** particularly lead and copper. Lead and its compounds are toxic to both men and women and have been associated with sterility, period problems, impotence, sperm damage, miscarriages, stillbirths, and increased infant deaths. Lead levels in drinking water in some areas remain unacceptably high. We all need a certain level of copper in our bodies, but too much in water which flows through copper pipes may deplete essential zinc levels.

■ **Pharmaceuticals and chemicals:** a large number of medicinal drugs can have harmful effects, even if you are only handling rather than ingesting them. Anyone working on the manufacture of the contraceptive pill or anti-cancer drugs should be aware of the dangers. People who work in chemical and cleaning industries also come into contact with powerful chemicals. Pesticides and insecticides can also be potentially dangerous, and chemicals used in hairdressing and dry cleaning can have side effects on both a woman and her unborn child. The list of these dangerous substances is still increasing—every year it is thought that between 700 and 3,000 new industrial chemicals are introduced. Nobody knows for sure what effects they may have on the reproductive system.

■ **Computer terminals:** although there is no undisputed evidence to prove that radiation from computer screens is harmful, you might choose to take the extra precaution of fitting a radiation screen on your terminal, if possible. Make sure you take a break from the screen for at least 10 minutes in every hour.

WHAT CAN YOU DO TO HELP YOURSELF?

You may find it relatively easy to control your environment at home but what about the workplace?

■ If you are worried about reproductive hazards at work—or the effect something might have on your pregnancy—raise the issue with your employer. All products that are used at work must be supplied with information as to their safe use. If your employer can't answer your questions it should be possible to find out.

■ If you are concerned about passive smoking at work, raise the issue with your employer. You could suggest introducing a policy about smoking in the workplace. Try to enlist the support of colleagues at work who may welcome the idea of smoke-free zones.

■ **X-rays:** these may be harmful to the fetus during pregnancy, which is why it is important to have any investigations which require X-rays done before you get pregnant. Many countries lay down standards for women working in hospitals and laboratories.

Note: there is probably little risk to anyone passing through X-ray machines used for security checks.

■ **Dental work:** have a full dental check-up at this stage, too—a woman's gums get softer and are more vulnerable during pregnancy. Debate still rages about whether the mercury in amalgam fillings causes health problems or not. The British Dental Association says that while there is no danger from existing fillings, mercury can be released into the system when fillings are taken out for the teeth to be refilled.

Right: if you work at a VDU screen, you should take a break every hour.

SUMMARY

Preparing for pregnancy might sound like hard work—but deciding to have a baby is probably one of the most momentous decisions you will ever take in your life. And if a job is worth doing, it's worth doing well—for the sake of all three of you.

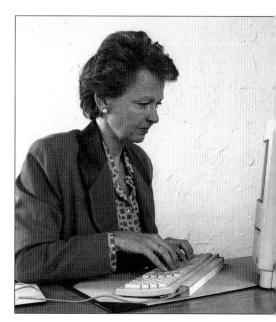

CHAPTER TWO

GOOD FOOD NATURALLY

Congratulations—you are going to have a baby. Now it is time to take those first steps as a mother, nourishing and nurturing the child-to-be. And you need to look after yourself, so you have the best chance of reaching the end of your pregnancy fit and healthy and prepared for the demands of caring for a new life.

A HEALTHY DIET

Eating a healthy diet when you are pregnant will not only keep you fit and well, but help your baby develop and grow. The exact relationship between maternal diet and fetal well-being is still a matter for some debate. Severe dietary restrictions are known to cause marked decreases in birthweights. Yet some experts argue that, in normal circumstances, a growing fetus takes what it needs, and if anyone's health is likely to suffer as a result of dietary deficiencies, it will be the mother's.

So where does that leave the average mom-to-be? As a general rule, women

Below: you should eat a varied, nutritious diet during pregnancy.

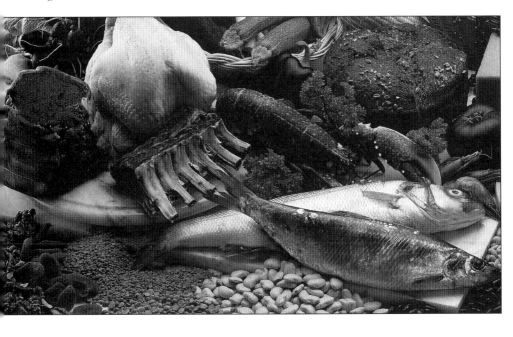

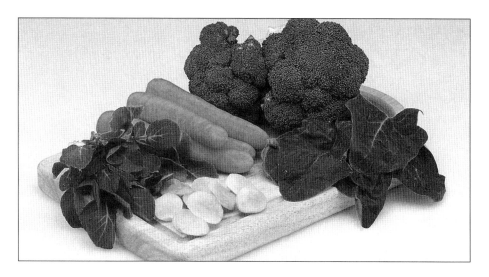

should never go on a diet when they are pregnant, unless it is on the advice of a doctor and under strict medical supervision. There again, it is probably not a wise idea to use your pregnancy as an excuse to double your food intake because you are "eating for two."

YOUR WEIGHT

Throughout your pregnancy, whenever you go for an antenatal appointment at a clinic or hospital you may be weighed, and a note taken of how much weight you have gained. Some doctors still firmly believe that women should not have a total weight gain of more than 28 pounds.

In fact, many women gain more or less: some may put on less than 14 pounds, others up to 42 pounds. On average, women tend to gain eight pounds in the first 20 weeks and about one pound a week after that. As you can see, most of the weight gain is likely to take place after the

Above: green vegetables, carrots, and apricots all contain vitamin A.

twentieth week and is the result not only of your baby growing, but also of your body storing fat to make breast milk.

Some doctors now believe that it is unnecessary to weigh all women routinely through their pregnancy or to advise them not to put on too much weight. They argue that, providing you are eating properly, a steady weight gain, with no sudden gains or losses, is more important than the actual amount you put on.

Too little weight gain is usually more of a worry than too much. But while this is reassuring for many women, it is also worth bearing in mind that if you do put on a lot of weight, you may suffer more tiredness in later pregnancy, you may have more stretch marks and you may find it harder to regain your figure in the future after the baby is born.

EATING DURING PREGNANCY

Of course, in the early days you may not feel like eating very much at all. Some women find that they develop an aversion to certain foods when they are pregnant. Others get odd cravings. And toward the end of the pregnancy, the baby may be taking up so much space, you could find it impossible to eat a proper meal at all.

It is probably best to listen to what your body is telling you, eat little and often if that works best, and use vegetables or fruit to snack on, rather than fatty or sugary foods.

Overall, you should aim to have a balanced diet, with a mixture of the four main food groups outlined below. Then you and your baby will both be getting all the nutrients you need.

Note: if you are on a restricted diet for health or other reasons, talk to your doctor.

FRUIT AND VEGETABLES

These provide vitamins and minerals along with fiber which helps digestion and prevents constipation. Try to have at least five portions a day. All the citrus fruits, strawberries and tomatoes are good sources of vitamin C. Bananas contain potassium as

Below: you need to eat plenty of fresh fruit, vegetables and whole grains.

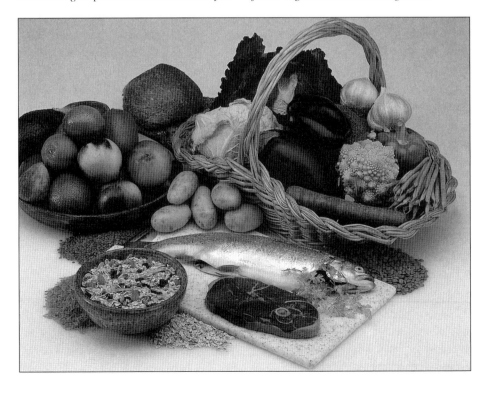

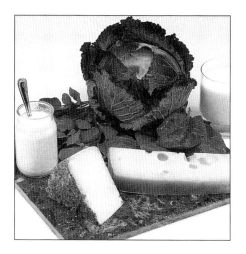

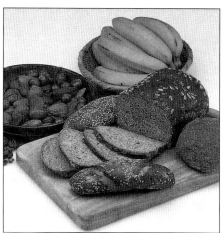

Above: green leafy vegetables and dairy products, such as cheese, milk, and yogurt, are good sources of calcium.

Above: vitamin B6 is found in bananas, whole-grain cereals, such as wholemeal bread, and nuts.

well as vitamins A, B6, and B12. Green leafy vegetables, soya beans, seaweed, and nuts all contain substantial amounts of Vitamin E. Wash fresh fruit and vegetables thoroughly to remove any traces of pesticides and chemicals. As many vitamins are water-soluble or destroyed by long periods of cooking, eat these foods raw when you can. If you do cook them, try lightly steaming or stir-frying.

The fresher the food the better. Food stored for any length of time, even in the refrigerator, loses vital nutrients. This is just as true for fresh fruit and vegetables as for pre-packed food with use-by dates.

STARCHY FOODS

Starchy foods, such as bread, potatoes, rice, pasta, and breakfast cereals, together with vegetables, should form the main part of

any meal. They contain complex carbohydrates which are satisfying, without being too high in calories, and they are also an important source of vitamins and fiber. Eat wholemeal bread and whole-grain cereals where possible.

LEAN MEAT, FISH, EGGS, BEANS AND LENTILS

These are good sources of protein, so eat some foods from this group every day. Some experts believe that pregnant women need more protein than usual, around two ounces a day. There are two ounces of protein in a two-ounce serving of chicken or fish.

DAIRY PRODUCTS (MILK, CHEESE, AND YOGURT)

These are good sources of calcium and other nutrients needed by your growing baby.

SHOULD YOU TAKE SUPPLEMENTS?

Some minerals are particularly important during pregnancy: folic acid, iron, and calcium. However, most women get the vitamins and minerals they need from the food they eat.

Women who are on a restricted diet may need extra vitamins and minerals—but no one should take supplements during pregnancy without taking medical advice.

■ **Folic acid** is the one important exception to the general rule. It is found in leafy green vegetables, whole-grain cereals, and eggs—but women who are trying to get pregnant are often advised to take a 0.4 milligrams tablet (400 micrograms) every day and to continue taking the supplement right up until they are 12 weeks pregnant.

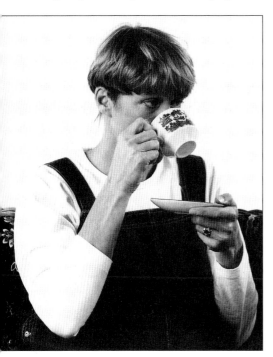

Even if you did not take folic acid before conception, it's worth starting as soon as you find out you are expecting a baby and continuing until you are 12 weeks pregnant. Folic acid supplements can help prevent neural tube defects in babies.

■ **Iron** is needed during pregnancy because the volume of blood circulating round your body increases. Extra iron is necessary to make hemoglobin for the increased number of red blood cells. The more hemoglobin your blood contains, the more oxygen it can carry to various tissues, including the placenta. If you are short of iron you will probably get very tired and may suffer from anemia.

Women used to be given iron supplements routinely, but now it is considered better if they get what they need from a normal diet. Iron is present in shellfish, lean red meat, whole grains, beans, seaweed, dried fruit and nuts, and green, leafy vegetables. You need vitamin C to help you absorb iron. Citrus fruit, tomatoes, broccoli, and potatoes are all good sources of this.

■ **Calcium** is essential for building healthy teeth and bones. Your baby's teeth and bones begin to form from weeks four to six. As your baby grows, so do your calcium requirements. Milk and dairy products are good sources. If you have an allergy to milk or other dairy products, you can still ensure that you get the calcium

Left: it is a very good idea to limit your caffeine intake and to opt instead for decaffeinated tea, coffee, and cola.

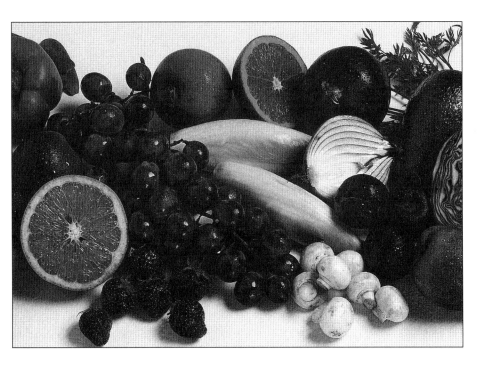

you need from your food. Fish with edible bones, e.g. sardines, bread, nuts, and green vegetables are also good sources.

Calcium cannot be absorbed efficiently without vitamin D. This is found in butter, milk, egg yolk and oily fish, but the best source is sunlight. So getting out and about in the fresh air will be good for you and your child.

FOODS TO TAKE CARE WITH

■ **Meat:** make sure raw meat does not come into contact with other food in the refrigerator and always wash surfaces and utensils after preparing it. Make sure you cook meat thoroughly so that there is no pink tissue or blood left. This will help you avoid catching toxoplasmosis, which can harm your baby.

Above: fresh fruit and vegetables are among the healthiest snacks—eat at least five portions a day.

■ **Fruit, vegetables, salads:** wash thoroughly to get rid of any soil which may contain toxoplasma.
■ **Eggs:** cook until the whites and yolks are solid to prevent the risk of salmonella. Avoid foods that may contain raw egg, e.g. home-made mayonnaise or mousse.
■ **Pâté and ripened soft cheese:** some physicians may advise you not to eat soft cheeses as well as blue-veined cheeses and those made from goat's or sheep's milk. These carry the risk of listeria infection, and although listeriosis is rare, even the mild form of the illness can cause miscarriage, still birth or severe illness in a newborn.

■ **Liver and liver pâté or sausage:** avoid as they contain a lot of vitamin A, and too much could harm the baby.

■ **Chilled and frozen foods:** make sure these are cooked thoroughly until they are piping hot.

■ **Drinks:** milk should be pasteurized. It is best to limit your intake of drinks containing caffeine. These include tea, coffee, and colas. There may be a slight risk that too much caffeine could affect the baby's birth weight. Try decaffeinated coffee, fruit juice, or mineral water instead.

When it comes to alcohol, research shows that heavy or frequent drinking can seriously harm a baby's development. Doctors disagree on the advice they give about light or occasional drinking during pregnancy—there is no evidence that this will cause any harm but to be on the safe side you might consider stopping altogether or having no more than one or two units of alcohol once or twice a week.

A unit is the equivalent of a half-pint of ordinary-strength beer or cider; a single measure of spirit; or a small glass of red or white wine.

FOODS TO CUT DOWN ON

There are two groups of foods which you can safely cut down on.

■ **Sugar and sugary foods**
These include candy, cookies, desserts and sugary drinks. Sugar contains "empty" calories—although these calories can give you energy, they don't provide any of the other nutrients the body needs. Sugar also increases the risk of tooth decay. If you feel the need for something sweet, reach for the fruit bowl, not the cookie jar.

■ **Fats and fatty foods**
Some fat is essential for health, but most of us eat more fat than we need. It is very high in calories and too much increases the risk of heart disease. So avoid fried foods, choose fish or chicken in preference to red meat and trim off any excess skin or fat. Choose low-fat dairy products when possible—skimmed or semi-skimmed milk, low-fat yogurt, half-fat hard cheese.

WHAT ELSE TO AVOID?

■ **Smoking:** if you smoke, then stopping now will be one of the most important things you can do for your baby. When you smoke cigarettes, carbon monoxide and nicotine pass into your bloodstream and as a result your baby gets less oxygen. This means it cannot grow as well as it should. Babies born to mothers who smoke tend to weigh less than other babies. They may have more problems during and after labor and are more prone to infection. They are more likely to be born prematurely, with all the additional breathing, feeding, and health problems this can bring.

■ **Drugs:** some can harm your baby. Even some over-the-counter medicines and prescribed drugs may cause problems. If you take regular medication, get your doctor's advice as soon as you think you may be pregnant.

Opposite: a healthy diet provides essential nutrients for you and your baby.

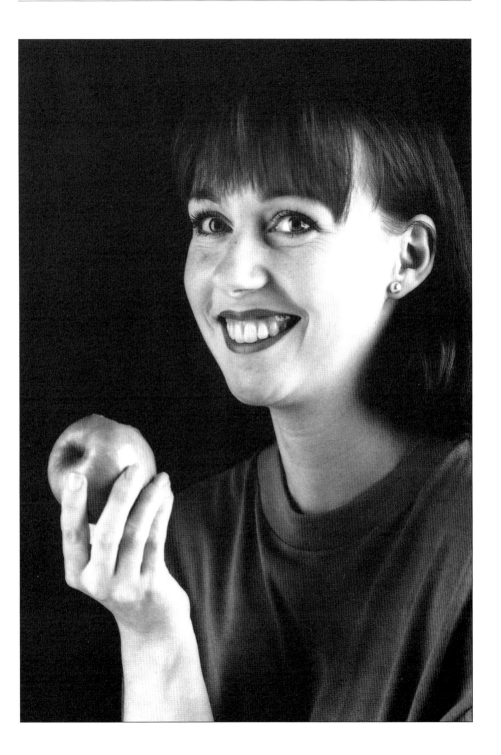

GET FIT FOR PREGNANCY

W e all need exercise: it improves the circulation, tones up muscles, strengthens our bones, keeps joints supple, and aids good posture. Exercise can help us stay mentally fit, too— it helps relieve stress and creates a feeling of well-being.

That's why exercise should be part of your pre-pregnancy planning. If you are fit and active when you embark on pregnancy, then you will find it easier to handle the demands that will be made on your body over the next nine months.

Besides, labor is not called labor for nothing: it can be very hard work. However, the fitter you are during your pregnancy, the better you will be prepared for childbirth. You are more likely to have a normal labor and to get back into shape after your baby is born.

INCREASE YOUR EXERCISE

■ Try to establish a pattern of taking regular exercise well before you conceive. If your lifestyle is not a very active one, make changes gradually. Aim to be a little more active every week as your strength and stamina increase.

■ Don't forget that everyday chores can be

Right: most women can carry on with their usual exercise routines in pregnancy.

a good way of keeping fit. Changing the beds, washing the kitchen floor or working in the garden are tasks that may have to be done anyway, so make them part of your activity plan.

■ Making small lifestyle changes can also help increase your fitness, and are easily incorporated into everyday routines. Stop taking easy options: use the stairs instead of the elevator; walk up escalators; walk to the next bus stop; leave the car at home for local trips.

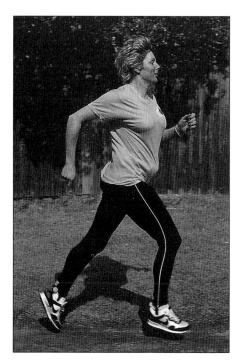

■ As well as this, you could go swimming, play tennis, cycle, take a brisk walk, or even dance along to your favorite CD. Choose something you enjoy and which fits into your lifestyle—that way you will be more likely to stick to it.

HOW MUCH EXERCISE?

Your aim should be to build up to doing half an hour of moderate-intensity physical exercise on five days of the week. Research has shown that this is the level of activity that significantly improves health.

Moderate exercise is the kind that leaves you with a warm, rosy glow, and slightly out of breath. Your heartbeat will be raised but you won't be sweating or panting. So you don't have to take up jogging or join an aerobics class to reap the health benefits of exercise—but if you do go to classes, make sure the leader is properly qualified, or you may end up doing more harm than good. And don't get carried away—women who exercise excessively often find that their periods stop altogether.

Once you are pregnant, provided you are in good health and have no previous history of miscarriage or premature labor, there is no reason why you shouldn't continue most sports or exercise routines as long as you feel comfortable. That said, most doctors advise against sports that are dangerous or especially vigorous.

■ **Swimming** is particularly beneficial during pregnancy. Not only is it relaxing (especially in the later months, when the illusion of being weightless is almost

> ### EXERCISE RULES
>
> ■ Whatever form of exercise you choose, start gradually and slow down comfortably.
> ■ Never go on until you feel exhausted and always stop if you feel any pain.
> ■ Make sure you drink plenty of fluids and avoid any strenuous exercise in hot weather.
> ■ If you are not sure whether it is wise to do something or not, check with your doctor.

miraculous) but it is one of the best all-round types of exercise.

Even non-swimmers can join aquarobic or water exercise classes for pregnant women. To find out if any are held in your area, check at your local library, gym, health club, or swimming pool. Water exercise can have a gentle toning effect on your muscles, help build up your strength and improve flexibility. However, as a safety precaution, always make sure someone is with you when you swim or exercise in water during pregnancy.

■ **Cycling** is another sport where something else—the bicycle—takes your weight while you build up your fitness. **Note:** if you were not very active before your pregnancy, don't suddenly rush into anything. You may not feel like doing very much, anyway, in the first three months when many women often feel sick or tired—but any amount of exercise is better than nothing. Just going for a walk can help improve your fitness.

WHEN TO START EXERCISING

■ Some doctors suggest that it is best to wait until you are past your twelfth week before you start any exercises, unless you are already accustomed to doing yoga or working out. The sooner you start after that the better, although it is never too late to gain some benefit.

■ Take it easy at first, trying out just a few examples, and gradually build up as your body gets used to the positions. As you loosen up and lose any stiffness, the exercises will feel more comfortable, but if individual ones feel wrong for you, leave them out. Listen to what your body is telling you. This is not a competition and it should be a pleasurable experience, not a painful one.

■ Always wear something loose that will not restrict your movements.

■ You need quite a large floor or wall space for some of the exercises, so choose part of a room that is free of furniture.

■ Try to find a time when you can be quiet and uninterrupted.

■ However tired you may feel, you will probably find it most beneficial to exercise either first thing in the morning or in the evening. It may seem a contradiction, but the exercises can give you added energy to cope with a busy day ahead, or help you to relax and sleep at the end of one.

■ Whatever time of day you choose, it is best not to eat a large meal beforehand.

Below: stretching exercises will help you loosen up. If you are already very fit, you can continue with gentle running during pregnancy (opposite).

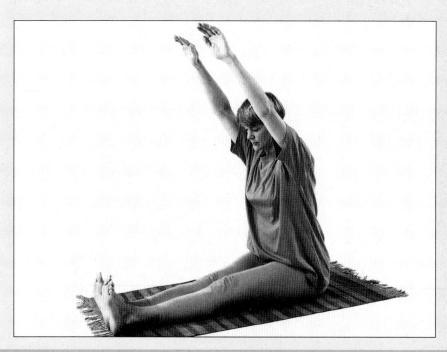

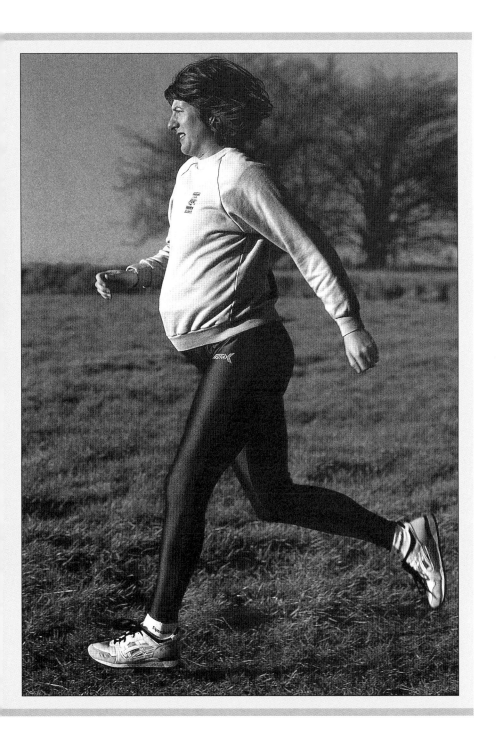

PELVIC FLOOR EXERCISES

One set of exercises all women should do— especially during pregnancy—is the pelvic floor exercises. The pelvic floor muscles support everything within the pelvic cavity, including the uterus, the bladder, and the rectum. During pregnancy, the pelvic floor is under extra stress so the muscles should be exercised several times a day.

If you are not sure how to locate these muscles, one of the ways to discover them and find out how they work is to sit on the toilet, start urinating and then, towards the end of the stream, try to stop the flow. Then finish emptying your bladder. (Don't try this if you have a urinary or kidney infection.)

The pelvic floor muscles are interconnected and work as a complete unit. Some of the muscle fibers can work strongly over long periods, while others can only work in short bursts. One of the most effective ways of exercising the pelvic floor muscles is to use a combination of slow pull-ups and fast pull-ups.

SLOW PULL-UPS

■ A slow pull-up should take about 10 seconds. Close up your back passage as if you were trying to prevent a bowel movement, draw in your vagina as if you were gripping a tampon, and your urethra as if you were trying to stop a flow of urine.

■ Start counting up to ten in your head (one—two—three—four) as you squeeze and lift. Now squeeze and lift harder (five—six—seven), then again (eight—nine—ten). Then relax. If you can't manage this to a count of ten, do it for as long as you can.

FAST PULL-UPS

■ A fast-pull up is exactly as it sounds: a quick lift and squeeze, then letting go.

■ Ideally, you should do five to ten slow pull-ups, followed by five to ten fast ones, as a set several times a day.

Below: during pregnancy it is important to exercise the pelvic floor muscles.

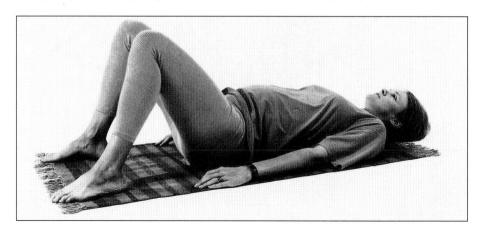

RELAXATION

In order for one set of muscles in the body to work, the opposite set has to relax. You can use this fact to carry out a sequence of movements to take your body away from a posture of tension to one where it is at ease and relaxed.

1 Start by lying quietly on your back with your legs slightly apart and your hands by your side. Some women— particularly in the later months of pregnancy—find that lying on their back can make them feel faint. If this happens to you, or if you feel uncomfortable, find an alternative position. You could lie on your side, your head on a pillow, with your top leg bent and supported by another pillow.

Alternatively, you could sit up against a wall, so that your back is straight and supported. Cross your ankles, keep your feet as close to you as possible, and let your knees drop as close to the ground as is comfortable. Alternatively, you could simply relax in a chair.

Close your eyes. Start with your shoulders, pulling them down toward your feet, then stop pulling. Notice how they have become relaxed.

Now move on to your arms. Push your elbows out and open—then stop pushing. Register the way in which your arms now feel relaxed.

2 Now your hands. Stretch your fingers so that they are long and straight—then

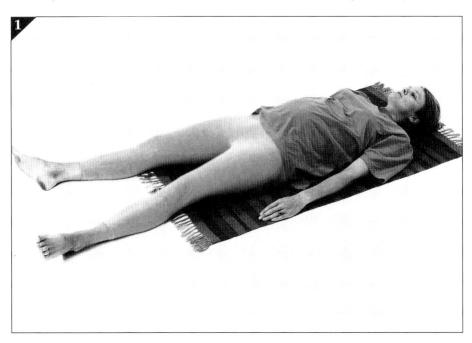

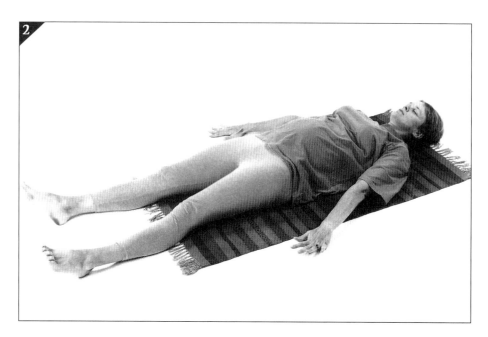

stop stretching. Notice how they are now loosely curled and relaxed.

Next, move on to your hips. Tighten your buttocks and press your knees out sideways. Now stop doing it. Register the relaxed feeling in your hips.

3 Move down to your legs. Lift your heels, then stop lifting. Feel how comfortable your knees and thighs feel.

4 Press your feet down and away from you, then stop. Notice how your feet are dangling on the ends of your legs. Press your body into the floor or the support behind you—and stop pressing. Register the sensation of relaxation you feel in your abdomen.

Do the same with your head. When you stop pressing, notice how relaxed your neck and upper shoulders have become.

Lastly, move up to your head. Drag your lower jaw down, then stop doing it. Notice how comfortable it feels when your upper and lower sets of teeth are both resting, slightly apart.

Stretch your lips sideways in a slight smile, pout forward very quickly and then stop doing it. Notice how pleasant it is when your lips are just lightly touching each other. Raise your eyebrows, then stop raising them. Imagine someone smoothing away the lines of tension on your forehead.

Now start listening to the pattern of your breathing, without disturbing it. Try to let your mind go as limp as your body. Feel the tension draining out of your body, into the floor. Imagine yourself getting heavier and heavier.

Begin to breathe in through your mouth and out through your nose. Breathe out fully, then pause until you feel the urge to

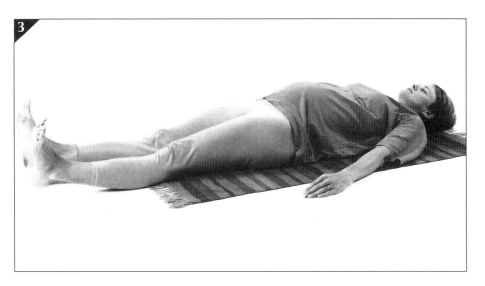

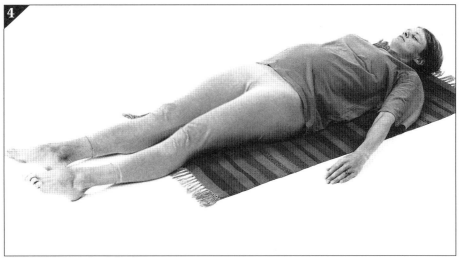

breathe in again. Let your stomach sink in as you breathe out and then expand again as you breathe in.

Concentrate on the "out" breath and let breathing in come naturally. Continue to pause between each breath. After a while, return to your normal breathing, in and out through your nose. Imagine something peaceful or beautiful, picture it in your mind, and focus on it. Enjoy the feeling of utter calm for a while.

Come back slowly. Wriggle your hands and feet. When you are ready, open your eyes and sit quietly for a while. Stretch, if you feel like it, yawn and then slowly start to move again.

OTHER EXERCISES

You may also like to try the following exercises. Two words of warning, however, before you start exercising.

1 Don't do anything while lying flat on your back if it makes you feel dizzy.

2 Stop at once if you feel any pain in your symphysis pubis—the joint between the two pubic bones at the front of the pelvis.

EXERCISE 1

Pelvic rocking and circling can tone up the abdominal muscles.

1 Lie on a flat, firm surface with your knees bent and your feet flat.

2 Pull your stomach muscles in and press the cheeks of your bottom together while you breathe out through your mouth. Then release the muscles as you gently rock your pelvis forward, and breathe in deeply through your nose.

3 Don't make the sequence too hurried or jerky, or the movement too exaggerated, and repeat it for as long as you feel comfortable.

Variations

■ You can kneel on the floor with your arms folded on the seat of a stool or chair. Circle your pelvis round to the left ten times. Then repeat in the opposite direction.

■ Another variation is to sit astride a chair with a high back, resting your arms on a pillow on the chair-back. This lifts your shoulders and takes the pressure off your ribs. Then rock your pelvis gently forward.

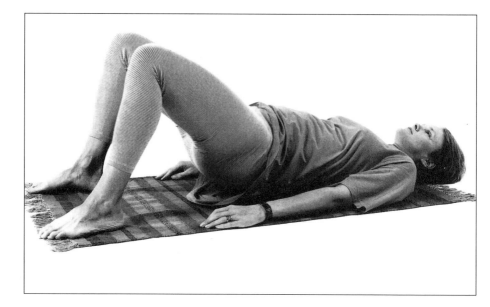

EXERCISE 2

This loosens the hip joints and helps stretch tight inner thigh muscles. Once you are used to it, it can be a very comfortable sitting position.

1 Sit up straight, on the floor, and bring the soles of your feet together as close to your body as possible. Clasp your toes or ankles with your hands to help you lift your spine. Another tip is to put a rolled-up towel under your coccyx.

You can also put your hands on the outside of your knees and push your knees against your hands to stretch the inner thigh muscles.

2 Next, interlock your fingers and stretch your arms out straight ahead of you, palms facing outward.

3 Keeping your arms stretched, inhale and raise them above your head. Don't hollow your back or push your ribs out. Hold for a moment, then exhale as you bring your arms down. Toward the end of your pregnancy this can feel wonderful as it opens up the body, giving the baby more space and you more room to breathe.

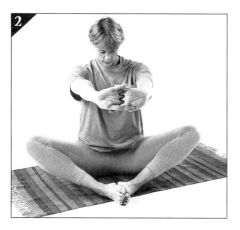

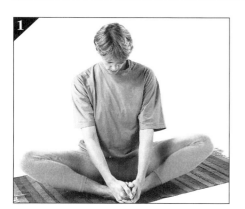

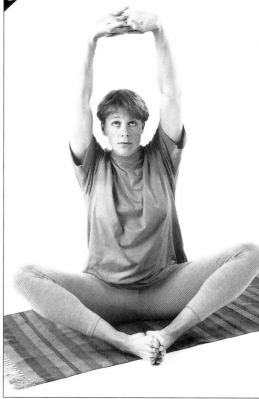

EXERCISE 3

This exercise will relax your back.

1 Kneel on the floor with your knees as wide as possible, your ankles turned out and your toes pointing toward each other. Sit between your feet if you can, or, alternatively, sit on your heels. Keep your back straight and bring your shoulder blades back and down to open your chest.

2 Move gently forward, keeping your bottom down and your arms straight, until your palms are flat on the floor. You should feel a stretch in your groin. Hold this position, breathing deeply, then slowly come up to a kneeling position.

3 If you cannot feel a stretch, go further down to rest on your elbows, but make sure you do not bend your back. Get your partner to check you are doing this correctly, or work in front of a mirror.

Note: if you still can't feel a stretch, you can slide your arms forward and lie flat. Don't force it. The aim is to feel the pull in your groin, not to get as low as possible.

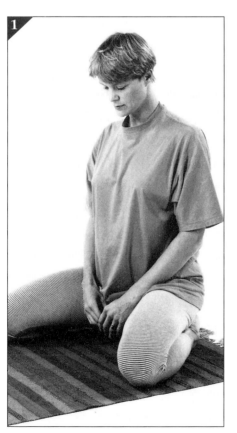

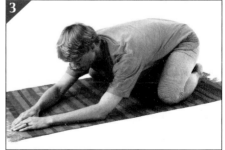

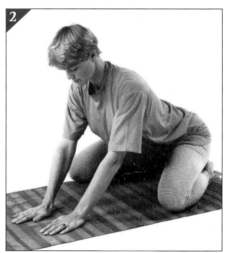

EXERCISE 4

This exercise loosens the shoulders and the top of the spine.

1 Sit on the floor with your knees up in front of you and apart. Stretch your right arm above your head.

2 Bend it at the elbow and reach down behind your back.

3 Stretch your left arm out to the side, bend your elbow behind you and try to clasp your right hand. Hold this position for a minute, then reverse.

Note: if you can't make your fingers meet when doing this exercise, use a scarf to hold on to.

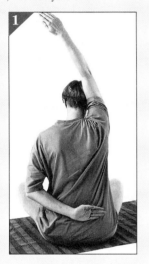 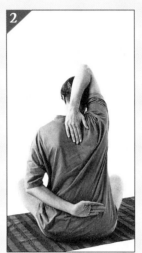 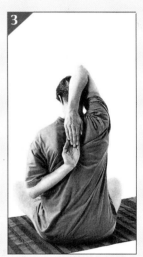

EXERCISE 5

This exercise stretches your inner thigh muscles.

1 Sit down sideways against a wall so that the side of your bottom is touching it. Swivel round so that, as you lie flat on your back, your bottom remains in touch with the wall and your legs are in the air. Bend your knees as if you were squatting and rest your feet against the wall. Lift your arms straight over your head.

2 Straighten your legs, keeping them together and hold this for a few seconds until you are used to the position.

3 Let your legs drop apart, sliding down the wall. Stretch your ankles and point your toes in toward your body.

4 The stretch in your inner thighs might feel uncomfortable at first. Hold the position for a minute or two, breathing deeply. Massage the inner thigh muscles with your hands, if it helps.

5 The best way of getting up afterwards is to roll slowly onto your side, pause for a second or two, and then go on to your hands and knees.

EXERCISE 6

This exercise mobilizes your back and strengthens your abdominal muscles.

1 Kneel on all-fours. Blow out and arch your back like a cat by tucking in your abdominal and buttock muscles so that your pubic bone moves forward. Hold the position for a few seconds.

2 Gently relax your muscles so that your back is flat again. Don't allow your lower back to hollow. Repeat the movement ten times.

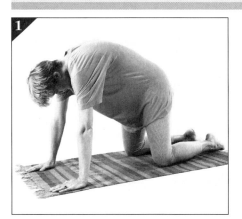
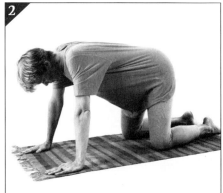

IMPORTANT

■ Whatever exercises you choose to do, always make sure that you start off with the relaxation sequence and then allow yourself time for another winding-down, relaxing session at the end.

■ Get into a comfortable position and allow yourself to be perfectly calm and relaxed. Close your eyes. Visualize every part of your body getting heavier and heavier, sinking down, down. With each breath out, relax a little more.

■ When it is time to come out of this relaxed state don't be in a hurry to sit up. Open your eyes. Become aware again of sounds, sensations. You may want to stretch gently. Move slowly. If you are on your back, roll to your side before getting up on to all-fours, and then into a sitting position.

■ Learning to relax like this is one of the most useful skills you will ever acquire. It will certainly help you cope with the stresses that can come with pregnancy and it will stand you in good stead when you go into labor. It will stop you wasting energy by tensing up in reaction to the power of your contractions and will help you disperse any stress and anxiety that might slow down the process of childbirth.

TONING AND STRENGTHENING EXERCISES

There are other exercises that are useful during pregnancy. These are not the vigorous "feel-the-burn" type, popular at many keep-fit classes, but gentle, toning, stretching movements. Many are adaptations of yoga postures, but you need never have practiced yoga to do them. You may wish to join a special yoga or exercise class for pregnant women, as it can be helpful to have a teacher explaining the movements and correcting you when necessary. To find out whether there are classes in your area, check at your local library or antenatal clinic.

If you can't get to a class, there are a number of books and videos available to help you follow a gentle exercise program at home. Some simple exercises are also suggested later in this chapter. However, if you have a chronic back problem, or if you have had any complications in this or in any previous pregnancies, such as a history of miscarriage or a Shirodkar (cervical) stitch, check with your doctor first.

TESTING FOR SEPARATION OF THE ABDOMINAL RECTUS MUSCLES

In late pregnancy it is quite common for the rectus muscles (which run straight up and down the abdomen) to separate. This is painless, but can lead to backache. To check for separation, lie on your back with knees bent and feet flat on the floor, hip distance apart. Place your hands on your abdomen as shown below, inhale, and lift your head and shoulders slightly, resting your chin on your chest. If there is separation you will feel the flesh bulging between the muscles. Post-natal exercises will close the gap.

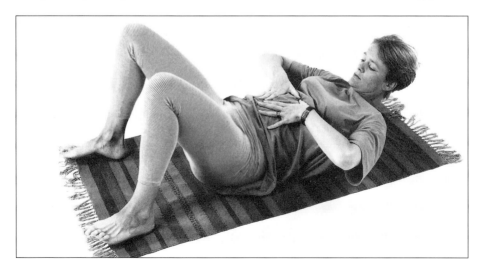

TUMMY STRENGTHENER

1 Lie on the floor with knees bent and slightly apart, feet flat on the floor. Lift your head and shoulders slightly off the floor and then reach out with your left hand and try to touch your right knee.

2 Lower yourself to the floor and repeat on the other side. If wished, you can use a cushion to support your head and shoulders when performing this exercise.

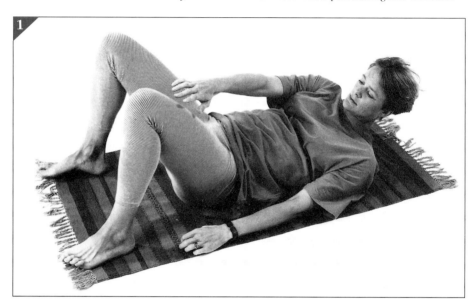

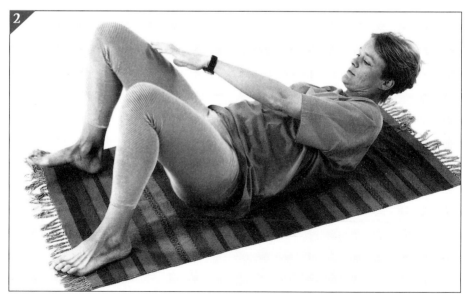

ABDOMINAL TONER

Lie on the floor with feet hip distance apart and knees bent. Cross your arms, exhale, and raise your head and shoulders, rolling up slowly. Hold for a count of three, pulling in your abdominal muscles. Inhale and lower your head and shoulders.

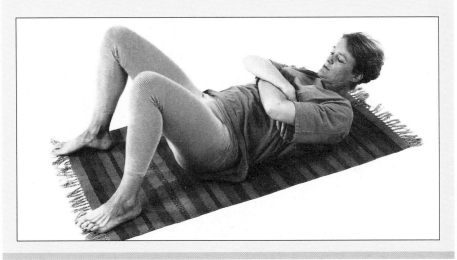

FOOT ROTATIONS

1 Sitting cross-legged on the floor, take your right knee in both hands and lift your leg off the floor.

2 Rotate it slowly in a large circle, pointing your toes on the up movement. Continue with toes down on the down movement. Repeat with the other leg.

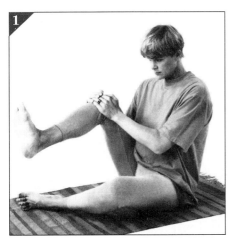

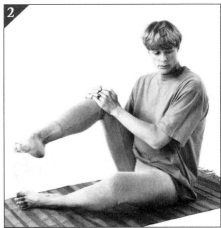

HEAD ROTATIONS

1 Sit down cross-legged with your hands resting lightly on your knees. Roll your head forward until your chin is resting on your chest.

2 Roll your head to one side and then round to the back.

3 Now roll your head round to the other side and then come full circle to the front. Repeat the head rotation in the other direction.

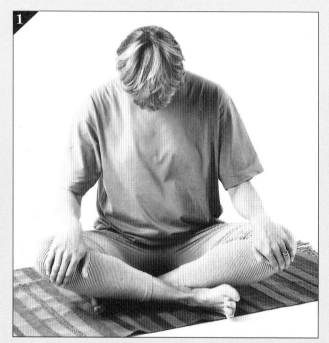

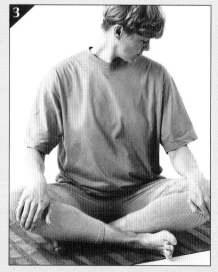

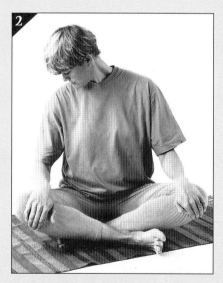

BRIDGING

1 Lie flat on the floor with some cushions under your head, arms at your sides, and your feet raised off the floor, resting on a box or a stool.

2 Pull in and tighten your buttocks and pelvic floor muscles. Slowly lift your lower back off the floor, keeping your back straight. Hold for a count of ten, then lower yourself slowly to the floor.

Note: bridging is particularly good for exercising the pelvic floor, buttocks and abdominal muscles.

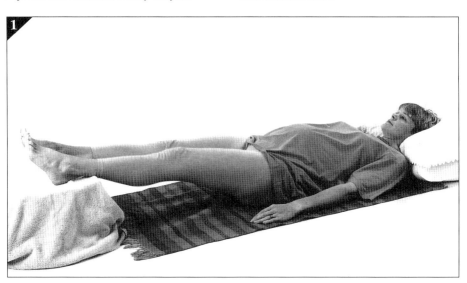

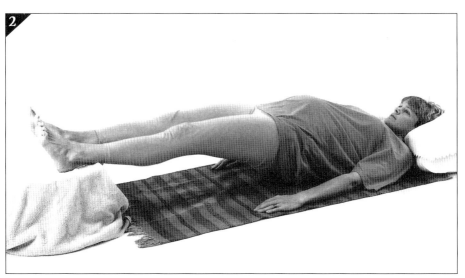

BUST STRENGTHENER

1 Stand with feet hip distance apart and raise your arms at 90 degrees to your body, bending your elbows.

2 Bring your arms into the center to touch at shoulder level with palms together. Inhale and open your arms again.

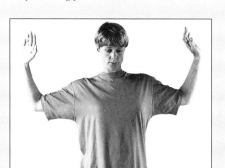
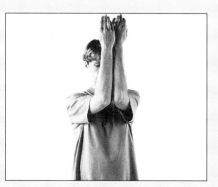

UPPER ARM TONERS

1 Stand with feet hip distance apart, arms crossed at shoulder level across your chest.

2 Inhale and throw open your arms as wide as possible. Exhale and cross them again. This strengthens upper arm muscles.

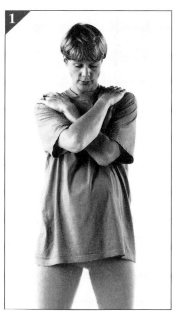
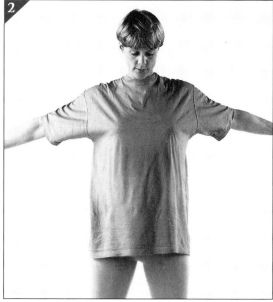

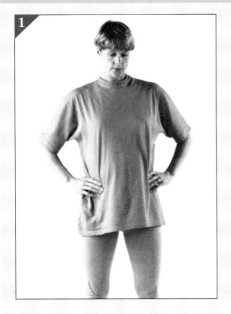

WAIST FIRMER

1. Stand with feet hip distance apart and your hands resting lightly on your hips.
2. Keeping your back straight, bend over slowly to one side from the waist only.
3. Now bend over to the other side. Come back slowly to the center.

Note: be sure only to lean over as far as feels comfortable, especially in the later months of your pregnancy when your "bump" is bigger. None of the stretches and exercises featured in this chapter should be uncomfortable or painful. If an exercise starts to hurt, then stop immediately.

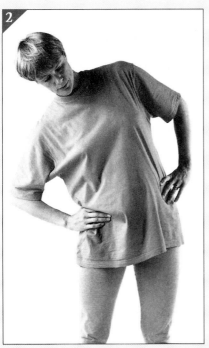

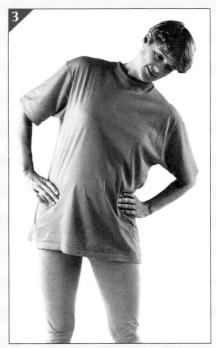

CHAPTER FOUR

STAY HEALTHY NATURALLY

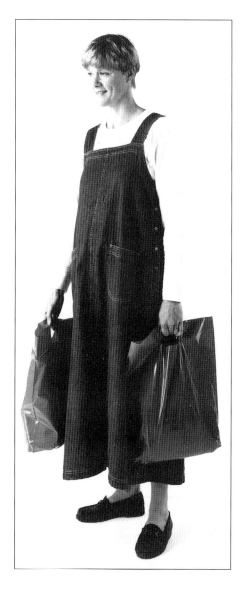

In romantic novels women glow their way through pregnancy, looking and feeling radiant. Real life is rarely like that. After all, your body undergoes all kinds of changes during these nine months and there may well be times when you feel tired and low.

The best way to look after yourself is to eat healthily, stay fit and supple, and make sure you have enough rest and relaxation. But there are also some specific things you can do to avoid or alleviate some of the common minor complaints of pregnancy.

You should not take drugs or medication when you are pregnant without first consulting your medical adviser. It is also advisable to take qualified advice before using any "natural" remedies or complementary medicine at home.

BACKACHE

As your ligaments soften and stretch to prepare for labor the strain this puts on your lower back and pelvis can cause backache. It is easier to take steps to prevent backache than it is to cure it once it has started.

Left: if you have to carry shopping, balance the weight evenly by using both hands. This helps prevent backache.

LIFTING

1 Avoid heavy lifting. Bend your knees when picking up objects. Keep your back straight whenever you are picking something up from the floor.

2 If you have to carry something heavy, hold it close to your body.

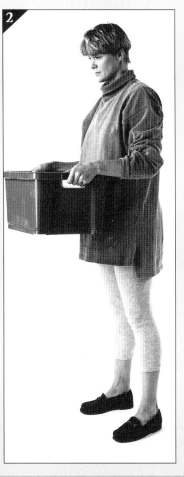

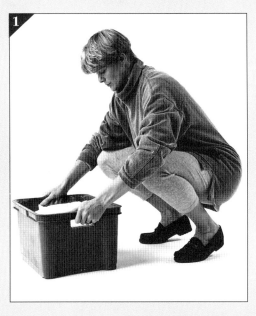

POSTURE

■ Think about your posture. Sit with your back straight and well supported. When you are standing, try not to let your back hollow. Tuck your buttocks in and relax your shoulders. Imagine you are a puppet on a string, being pulled up from the top of your head. You might consider taking some lessons in the Alexander technique.

■ A firm mattress can prevent and relieve backache. If your mattress is soft, you could put a board underneath it.

■ There are some exercises that can help relieve backache. If your upper back is the problem, try some shoulder rolls.

PELVIC ROCKING

■ This may also help. One way of doing this is an exercise called the angry cat.

■ Go down on all-fours. Keep the small of your back flat and, without moving your elbows or knees, tighten your stomach muscles and arch your lower back like a cat. Hold for a few seconds.

■ Relax, but do not let your back hollow. Repeat the sequence about ten times.

SHOULDER ROLLS

■ Rest your fingertips on your shoulders and circle backward with your elbows as if your arms were wings.

Note: if your backache is very severe, your doctor may be able to refer you to an

POSTURE

Good posture is very important in pregnancy, and the secret is to adjust it as the weight load of the baby increases so that you are well balanced with the baby's weight distributed evenly across your body. Your shoulders should be dropped to keep your spine straight and ease out tension. Stand straight and tall with buttocks tucked in (below left), not with your body thrust forward (below right).

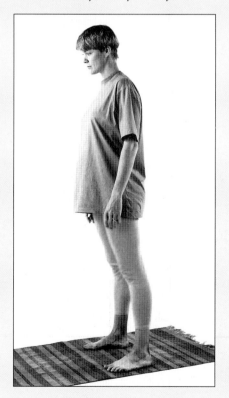 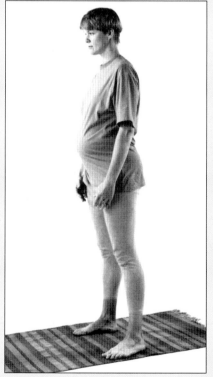

obstetric physiotherapist who will be able to advise you and may suggest some helpful exercises.

■ **Massage may also help**. Try lying on your side and get your partner to feel for the base of the tail bone between your buttocks. He should then press firmly with the heel of his hand, making small circular movements.

■ **One homeopathic remedy** is Kali Carbonica. Herbal decoctions of Ginger, Cinnamon, Lavender and Rosemary are also used to relieve backache. Add between one and two pints to a warm bath, and then have a soak.

■ **An osteopath or chiropractor** may also be able to offer a diagnosis and treatment.

Below: stop your system getting sluggish by eating plenty of fiber-rich foods, such as beans and lentils.

BREATHLESSNESS

This can be a nuisance in the later months when the baby is getting bigger. Acupressure, acupuncture, the Alexander technique, yoga, and naturopathy may bring some relief.

CONSTIPATION

■ Drink plenty of water and make sure you are eating fiber-rich foods, such as wholemeal bread, whole-grain cereals, fruit, vegetables, and pulses, e.g. beans and lentils. Exercise will help prevent your system getting sluggish. Some foods, such as prunes and figs, act as natural laxatives. Molasses does, too. The usual dose is about two teaspoons three times a day.

■ Many complementary therapies may help relieve this condition, including reflexology, aromatherapy, and homeopathy. Don't take over-the-counter laxatives without consulting your doctor.

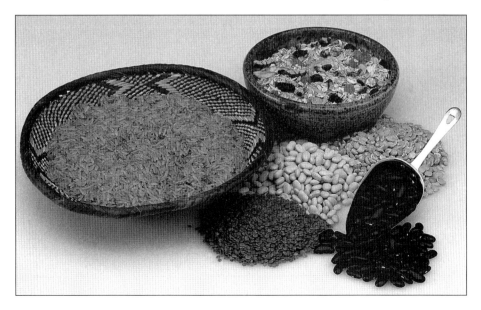

CRAMP

To avoid getting cramp in your calf muscles or feet you can do some regular, gentle exercises.

■ When sitting, try rolling your feet round in circles from the ankles or roll a bottle or rolling-pin back and forth with your feet.

■ If you are woken up with cramp in your calf, get your partner to grip your heel and push your foot up while pressing down on your knee with their other hand. If you are alone, push your foot hard against something firm like the bottom of the bed or a wall, stretching your ankle and pressing down on your own knee.

■ Homeopaths suggest various treatments, including arnica, cuprum metallicum, and nux vomica. Herbal teas, including those made from cramp bark or kelp, may also help. You could also try warm foot baths, with a few drops of Lavender oil.

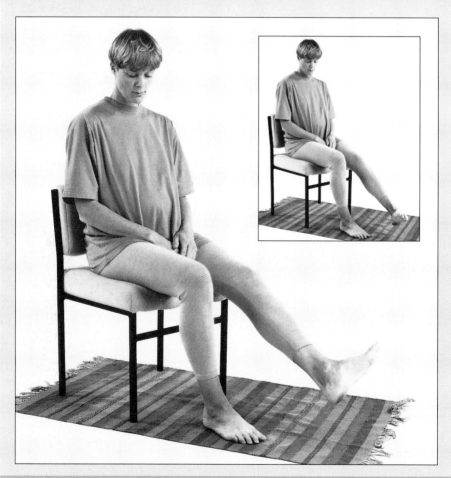

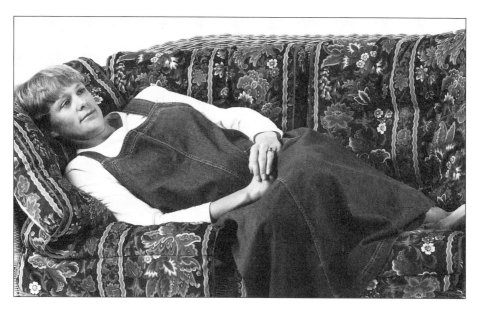

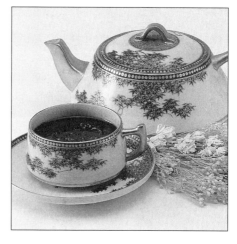

Above: extreme tiredness is a common symptom of early pregnancy. Do not fight fatigue but rest whenever you can. A cup of herbal tea (right) can be helpful in preventing indigestion.

FATIGUE

■ Many women are surprised at how tired they feel, particularly in the early months of pregnancy. Listen to the signals your body is sending you and rest when you can.

■ An aromatherapy massage may help you recharge your batteries, or you might like to add oils of Lavender, Rosemary, Frankincense or Thyme to your bath. Some oils must be avoided during pregnancy. Always seek qualified advice.

INDIGESTION AND HEARTBURN

■ Eating little and often may prevent the problem. Avoid highly spiced or fatty foods.

Sit up straight when you are eating as this takes the pressure off your stomach.

■ It may help to sleep well propped up, either by having plenty of pillows or by raising the head of your bed.

■ Don't take antacids before checking they are safe in pregnancy. Herbalists recommend Peppermint, Chamomile or Fennel tea. Milk and yogurt may relieve the symptoms of indigestion. Homeopathic remedies may also be prescribed.

INSOMNIA

Later on in pregnancy it can be difficult to get a good night's sleep. It may help to use pillows to get comfortable. Try lying on your side with a pillow under your stomach and another between your knees.

■ If you are woken up by the baby's movements it may help to get up and walk around for a little while to lull them back to a calmer mode.

■ Try some relaxation and breathing exercises. Some women find that herbal drinks, such as Chamomile tea, are helpful if taken before going to bed. Reflexology or acupuncture may also bring relief.

■ An aromatherapy massage at bedtime can be relaxing and may help you sleep. You could try putting a drop of Neroli oil on your pillow.

NOSE BLEEDS

These often occur during pregnancy because of the higher hormone levels and congestion which make it easier to damage the blood vessels in the nose.

■ You can prevent nose bleeds by stifling

Below: to help combat insomnia in the later months of pregnancy, lie with a pillow supporting your stomach and knees.

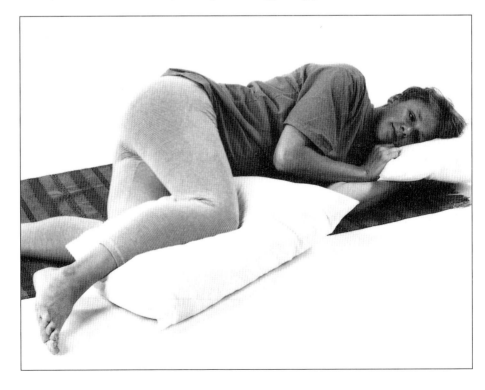

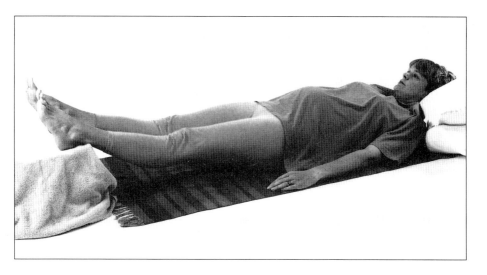

sneezes and blowing your nose gently. If you put a little petroleum jelly in each nostril at night you will stop your nasal passages getting cracked and dry.

Above: resting with your feet higher than your head for an hour a day, if possible, may help to prevent fluid retention and swelling in your ankles.

EDEMA

Fluid retention may cause your hands and ankles to swell a little. So try to avoid standing for long periods. If you have to stand, keep shifting from foot to foot, or move around a little, so that your calf muscles pump the blood and fluids back into the rest of your body.

■ Do some regular foot exercises—bend and stretch your feet up and down vigorously 30 times. Wear comfortable shoes and try to rest for an hour a day with your feet up higher than your heart.

■ Acupressure, acupuncture, massage, aromatherapy, naturopathy, and herbal or homeopathic remedies may help. Seek advice from a qualified practitioner or consult your doctor.

PILES

Piles—also known as hemorrhoids—are swollen veins which often occur during pregnancy because of the hormonal changes going on in your body.

■ Drinking plenty of water and eating a high-fiber diet will prevent constipation and you should also try to avoid standing for long periods. Regular exercise will help improve your circulation.

■ An ice pack may ease any discomfort and Cypress oil is said to shrink piles. Add a few drops to a large bowl of warm water and sit in it for as long as you feel comfortable. Ask your doctor, midwife, or complementary practitioner to recommend a suitable ointment to relieve pain or itching. Piles usually go soon after the baby is born.

PREGNANCY SICKNESS

Feeling nauseous is one of the earliest signs of pregnancy. Some women feel sick, some are sick—not just in the morning, but all day long. Most women find that the nausea disappears around weeks 12 to 14, but some are not so lucky.

■ Get as much rest as you can. Feeling tired can make the nausea worse. Give yourself time to get up slowly. Eat something like dry toast or a plain biscuit before you get out of bed.

■ Eat little and often during the day. Don't stop eating altogether.

■ Drink plenty of fluids. Some women find that carbonated water takes away the nauseous feeling.

■ Having a snack before you go to bed—however little you feel like it—may also make you feel less sick in the morning.

■ Some doctors think vitamin B6 can help, so it may be worth eating foods that are high in this vitamin, such as whole-grain cereals, wheatgerm and bananas.

■ Acupressure, acupuncture, herbal, and homeopathic remedies may help. The most commonly prescribed homeopathic remedy is ipecacuana, but other remedies may be more appropriate in individual cases. Herbalists often recommend Peppermint or Ginger.

■ Some women have been helped by using Sea-Bands, elasticated toweling bands with a small round plastic stud, worn on both wrists. Based on the Chinese principle of acupressure, the bands exert pressure on the points inside each wrist which are said to control the harmonization of the digestion and stomach. Sea-Bands are available from most drugstores.

SKIN AND HAIR CHANGES

Hormonal changes in your body will also affect your skin and hair. Your nipples will go darker and your skin color may deepen, either in patches or all over. Some women also develop a dark line running down the middle of their stomach. Most of these changes reverse themselves after the baby has been born.

■ Any marks will be made deeper by exposure to sunlight, so wear a hat to shield your face when you are out in the

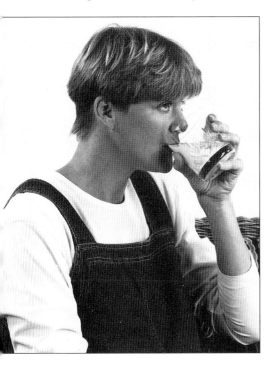

Left: keeping up your fluid intake, e.g. carbonated water, may combat nausea.

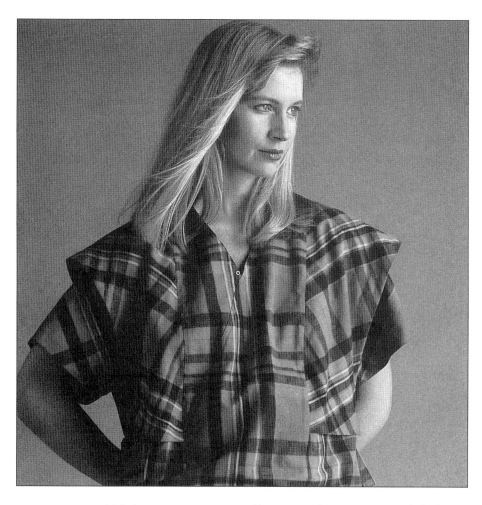

sun or use a very high-factor sunscreen.

■ Your hair may grow faster and may get greasier. You may have to switch to a different type of shampoo. Once the baby is born you may think you are losing a lot of hair—but you will only be losing the extra hair you gained in pregnancy.

STRETCH MARKS

Whatever some people claim, there is nothing you can do to be sure of preventing

Above: some fortunate women do look radiant throughout their pregnancy with glowing skin and healthy hair.

stretch marks. Some women get them, some don't, depending on their skin type. Some women's skin is simply more elastic than others, although you are more likely to get stretch marks if you put on too much weight.

■ Even so, there are steps you can take to minimize them. It helps if you keep your skin supple by regularly massaging your breasts, abdomen, and thighs with some cream or oil.

■ Special aromatherapy oils and herbal preparations are sold for this purpose, but even baby oil would do. Make sure you wear a well-supporting bra, even if this means buying several different ones as you progress through your pregnancy.

THRUSH

It is normal to have an increased vaginal discharge during pregnancy but if you start to itch or feel sore, you may have developed thrush. Pregnant women are particularly prone to thrush, which is caused by a yeast-like fungus, Candida albicans.

■ You can help prevent thrush from developing by wearing cotton underwear, rather than nylon ones. You should also avoid pantyhose and tight pants as they help to create the warm, moist conditions that thrush prefers.

■ Take extra care with personal hygiene: dry yourself thoroughly and always remember to wipe from front to back when you go to the toilet.

■ To relieve a mild attack of thrush, some women find that live natural yogurt, inserted into the vagina using a tampon, is sufficient. Others bathe the vaginal area with a solution of vinegar and water.

■ There are also homeopathic and herbal remedies for thrush. However, if your symptoms persist for longer than a week, despite any do-it-yourself treatment, you should see a doctor.

TEETH AND GUMS

When you are pregnant the margins of the gums around your teeth become much softer and spongier than usual and the hormonal changes in the body can cause any build-up of plaque to make the gums more inflamed. They may become swollen or bleed easily.

■ You can help to prevent any dental problems by brushing your teeth well, to remove all the plaque.

■ Avoid sugary drinks and foods.

■ Have a check-up at your dentist, but tell him that you are pregnant.

VARICOSE VEINS

During pregnancy some women develop varicose veins in their legs. Some get them in the vulva. Most types of varicose veins disappear within a few months of the birth.

■ To prevent varicose veins, try to avoid standing for long periods and don't sit with your legs crossed.

■ Try not to gain too much weight, as this will increase the pressure on your veins.

■ Any kind of exercise that helps the circulation is a good idea. This could be swimming, cycling, or walking. Do some foot exercises, too.

■ Support pantyhose may be useful. Put it on before you get out of bed in the morning.

■ A few drops of Cypress oil in your bath may help, too.

Opposite: gentle walking every day improves the circulation and helps to prevent varicose veins forming.

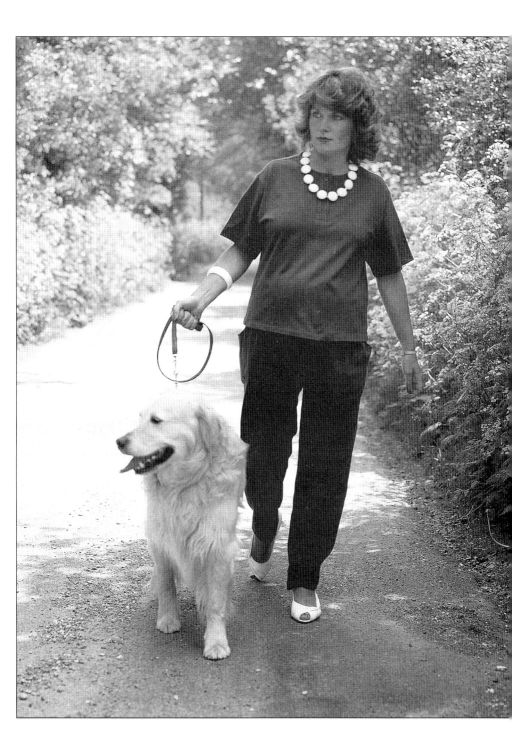

GET FIT FOR LABOR

B y the time you reach the later weeks of pregnancy you should be starting to think about getting ready for labor. Soon your uterus will have reached its highest point. The extra pressure on your stomach and lungs may make eating and breathing difficult and the extra weight that you are carrying around might make going out anywhere or doing anything feel like an uphill struggle.

Once your baby's head engages, you may get strange buzzing sensations in your pelvic region. It may even be uncomfortable to sit down. The extra pressure on your bladder may mean you make more frequent trips than usual to the bathroom. If you laugh or cough you may leak urine.

Above all, you may feel quite exhausted, yet when you try to sleep at night the baby keeps you awake, squirming and digging its knees and elbows into you.

DIET

Now is the time to take extra care of yourself. You should carry on eating a balanced diet to give you the energy and nutrients you will need to go though labor and delivery, even if this means eating little and often, rather than sitting down to full meals.

SLEEPING

If you are not sleeping well, try not to let it bother you. Relaxation or gentle exercise, a

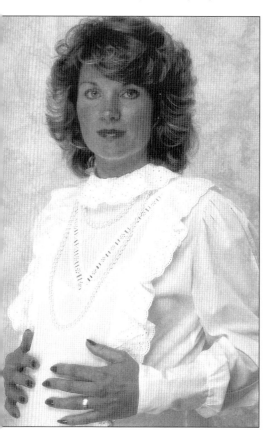

Left: the last weeks of pregnancy are a special time when you are looking forward to the birth of your baby. You can help prepare for labor by practicing your breathing and birth positions.

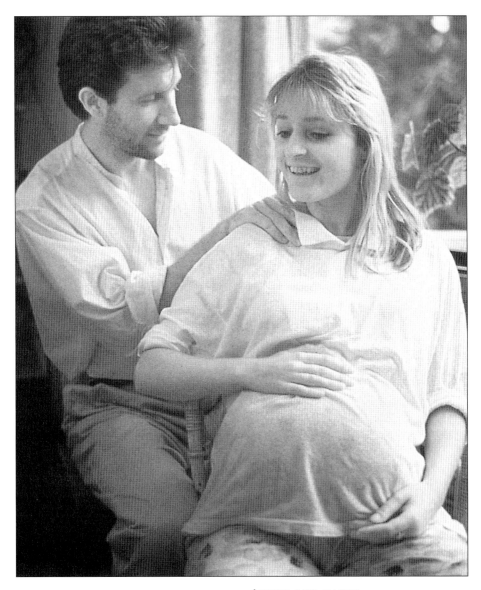

Above: the last weeks are a joyous time for you and your partner.

milky drink, or a warm bath before bedtime may help. Catch up on missed sleep by resting or taking naps during the day.

ACHES AND PAINS

If you are suffering from backache or any of the other minor complaints which can mar these last weeks, check back to Chapter Four to see if there is anything you can do to help yourself.

ANTENATAL CLASSES

At about eight to ten weeks before the baby is due, most women start attending antenatal classes. These are usually held once a week, either during the day or in the evening, and last one or two hours. Some classes are for women only, whereas others encourage partners to attend all or some of the sessions.

The kind and number of classes vary from area to area. Some classes may be run by midwives or local or national organizations, or by your own doctor. They may be held in health clubs, hospitals, surgeries, or health centers.

Most classes are run as group sessions. They generally aim to provide accurate and reliable information about pregnancy and

Below: antenatal classes encourage partners to share the experience of pregnancy.

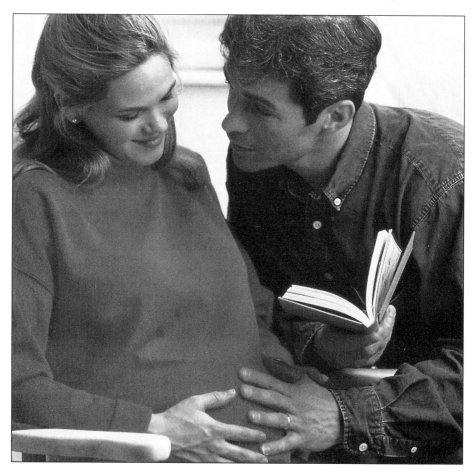

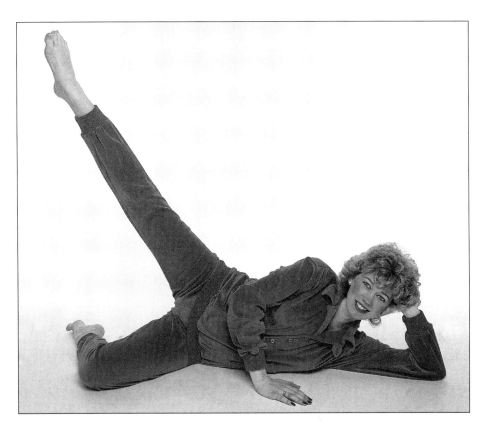

birth and the different experiences women will encounter. They can be a useful source of information about the kind of exercises that can keep you fit right up until the end of your pregnancy and will help you during labor. They can teach you relaxation techniques which will be useful before and after the birth, as well as specific breathing patterns which will help you cope during the first, second, and third stages of labor.

Classes should also give you a chance to find out about the choices available to you so that you can draw up your own birth plan. They may give you the opportunity to meet some of the professionals who will be

Above: you may do some strengthening and stretching exercises at antenatal classes.

involved in your care, and to ask questions and talk over any worries you might have. You will also be able to share your thoughts and feelings with other parents as well.

Attending antenatal classes can give you confidence. Of course, lots of women have babies without ever having been to one of these classes: giving birth is, after all, a natural event. But learning more about the process of childbirth can help you to understand your body so you can work with it during labor.

RELAXATION AND BREATHING TECHNIQUES

Two of the essential things you should learn at antenatal classes are relaxation and breathing techniques. If you are tense during labor your muscles contract and you hold your breath. This can slow things down, putting additional stress on you and your baby. It may also deprive you and your baby of some of the oxygen you both need. By tensing up in reaction to a contraction you waste valuable energy. The more exhausted you become, the more keenly you will feel any pain and the less you will feel in control.

Being able to relax when you need to—and not only when you feel in the mood to—is a useful skill to acquire. And now is the time to practice that skill so that when labor starts you will be able to keep a clear mind and respond to what is happening. There are some suggestions about relaxation on page 29. Antenatal teachers may have different techniques to suggest, such as touch relaxation.

TOUCH RELAXATION

■ This is a method in which you respond to a massage given to you by your partner or a friend. As they touch or stroke a part of your body you react to the pressure and warmth of their hands by relaxing the muscles there, and letting the tension go.

■ Choose a comfortable position, and breathe out, letting your muscles relax as you do so. Now contract one set of muscles—in your shoulders, for example. Feel the difference between the relaxed and the tense state.

■ As your partner puts his hands on your shoulders, and applies gentle pressure you should relax the muscles, with a sense of flowing out toward his touch.

■ It can be useful to practice touch relaxation in the last months of pregnancy as this is a technique which can be very

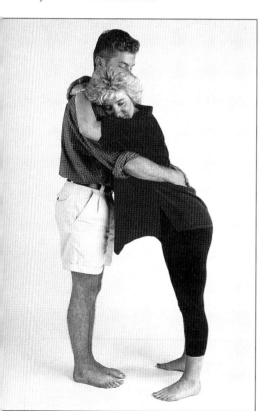

Left: let your partner help you relax instead of tensing up during contractions. This way you conserve your energy.

helpful in labor. Your partner learns to read your body language, so he can see when there is a build up of tension in you. During labor, if your partner notices your shoulders are getting tense, he can put a firm hand on them. He can stroke your arms or your legs.

■ Of course, you don't have to use touch relaxation to have a successful labor. When the time comes, some women find they do not want to be touched in this way at all. Even so, you will have to cope with physical examinations from a doctor or midwife, and exploring touch relaxation before the birth means you are teaching yourself to relax toward touch, rather than pulling away from it.

RELAXING IN LABOR

■ Learning to relax in response to pressure, rather than tightening up against it, may also be helpful when you find yourself in the throes of contractions and again when the baby starts to move down the birth canal. Instead of tensing up, you may be able to flow along with what is happening to you.

Below: as your partner learns to read your body language, he can help you stay in control through your labor.

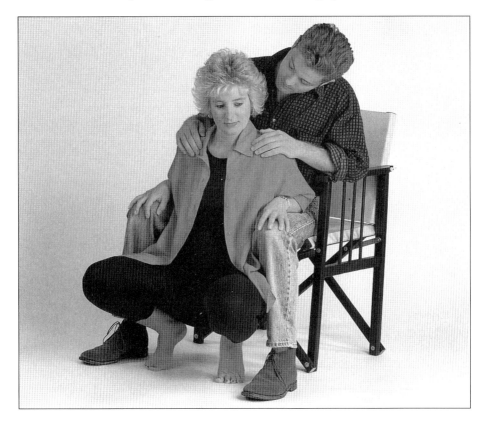

BREATHING TECHNIQUES

■ Just as there are many different ways of learning relaxation techniques, there are various breathing methods taught in preparation for labour. In practice the two go together. It's hard to relax properly if you are holding your breath, and it's hard to breathe properly for labor if you are not relaxed.

■ Breathing for labor usually involves learning to use different levels, the idea being to go up through the levels as contractions get stronger. For early contractions the first level of breathing will probably be adequate. As contractions get longer and stronger you will need to move up through the levels until you reach the peak, and then come back down again.

■ The idea of practicing your breathing well in advance of labor is to make it second nature, so that you can automatically adapt and go with the flow when the time comes.

■ Some people compare it to learning to drive a car: once you know how to use the brake and the accelerator you don't have to think about slowing down or going faster— your feet move automatically on the pedals depending on the traffic conditions that you experience.

■ Contractions can last from about 40 seconds to a minute-and-a-half once labor is established. They may be evenly paced, so that you know you will have a guaranteed rest period before the next one, or they may be all over the place. So when

PRACTICE YOUR BREATHING FOR LABOR

1 You can practice your breathing exercises in the position known as tailor sitting. Sit on a flat surface with your back straight and the soles of your feet pressed together. Now place both your hands on your abdomen and breathe in slowly through your nose. Exhale through your nose or mouth. Try to relax your abdominal muscles as you breathe out. You should be able to feel how these muscles respond during breathing by pressing lightly on either side of the abdomen as shown. As you inhale, your abdomen should move out—as you exhale, the muscles should be relaxed.

2 You can also practice this abdominal breathing sitting in a more conventional cross-legged position as shown.

3 It is useful to practice panting for dealing with the peak of a contraction when it is more difficult to relax. Quicker breathing in shallower breaths will help you surmount the pain and then ease down gradually into slower, more rhythmic breathing as the contraction subsides. Place your hand on your upper chest as you practice this panting and feel it moving. You may find it easier when you switch to this type of breathing to breathe in and out quickly two or three times, then sigh and pant again.

4 Now practice the routine of breathing through a contraction in a cross-legged position with your hands resting lightly on your knees. Try to feel your chest rising and falling and relax your abdominal muscles as you do so.

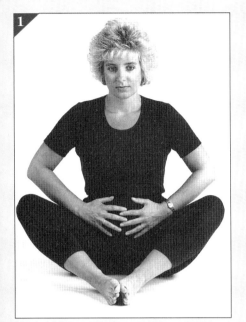

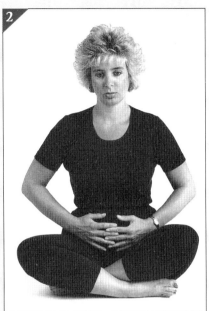

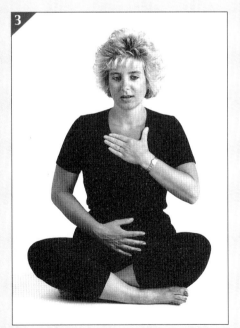

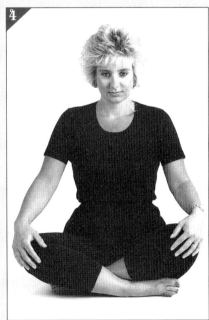

you are practicing your breathing you will just have to generalize.

■ For a long contraction towards the end of the first stage of labor you could start with ten seconds at the first level of breathing, 20 seconds each for levels two and three, and 30 seconds for the top level. Then do the same as you come down the scale.

■ **The breathing levels** get shallower as the contractions get harder. The idea is to lift your breathing to your upper chest, away from your uterus, freeing your stomach muscles to work with the stronger contractions. Focusing on your breathing can help you to remain calm and in control, as well as raising your pain threshold and conserving your energy.

■ **Level one** is a quite deep, full-chest breathing. Meet the contraction with a deliberate slow breath out. Continue to breathe slowly, in through your nose from down below your ribs and then out through your mouth.

■ **Level two** is higher up the chest. You can think of this as lifting your breathing above the contraction as if you were skimming the crest of a wave. Breathe lightly in and out through your mouth, putting the emphasis on the out breath as if you were blowing out candles.

■ **Level three** is the quickest, shallowest breathing to take you over the top of the strongest contractions. Some teachers suggest just mouthing the words "out, out" regularly and gently. If you concentrate on the "out" breath, breathing in will come naturally.

■ **Level four** is for the peak of the strongest contractions. If you mouth a song or count backwards from 50, you will be breathing without thinking about it, and taking your mind off the contraction. It is always best to pick something simple, so that it won't fly out of your head in the heat of the moment.

■ As the contraction begins to fade, the idea is to come back down through the levels, finishing with a long, slow in and

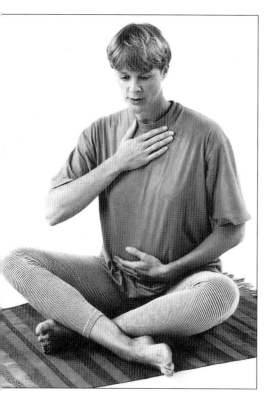

Left: as your pregnancy progresses, it is a good idea to practice your breathing in readiness for labor.

BREATHING FOR CONTRACTIONS

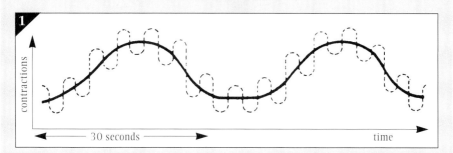

30 seconds   time

1 Breathing for gentle contractions before leaving for hospital. Breathe easily and rhythmically with the contractions—not too deep nor too fast. These contractions can be done while standing, lying down or bending over. Just try to relax into the contractions.

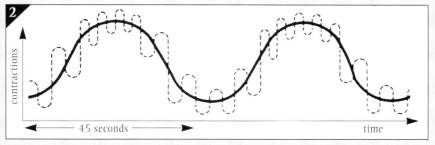

45 seconds   time

2 Further breathing as the contractions increase in strength. You will have to breathe faster and more shallowly in the upper chest at the peak of the contraction when relaxation becomes more difficult, maybe sitting in a comfortable chair.

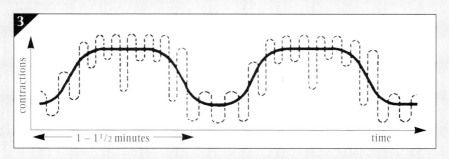

1 – 1 1/2 minutes   time

3 Breathing for the end of the first stage of labor when contractions become more intense and longer. Breathe in groups of three, in-out, in-out, in-sigh. It may help to lie on your side. You may feel you want to push. Panting may help if you are not yet fully dilated.

out cleansing breath. This resting breath helps you relax and lets everyone with you know that the contraction is over.

■ Once you have mastered the different levels, so that you can switch between them automatically, you will be able to use them in labor to suit yourself. You don't have to stick to a prescribed pattern. Some women can breathe up through the levels and down again. Others discard the first two levels early on.

TRANSITIONAL BREATHING

There is another type of breathing which can be very helpful during the transition stage of labor, when you are nearing the second stage but your cervix is not quite fully dilated. At this point you may feel you are not getting anywhere, you may feel sick or shivery, you may feel you want to start pushing, although you've been told it is too early. Transitional breathing can be a repetition of two blowing out breaths and then a pant: hoo, hoo, ha, hoo, hoo, ha.

One way of practicing your breathing is to get your partner to give you a "mock" contraction. He can squeeze your arm or ankle, first gently, then harder, while you

COMPLEMENTARY THERAPIES

Herbalists suggest that Raspberry leaf tea can help prepare the uterus for labor. Caulophyllum is a homeopathic remedy which is said to tone and relax the uterus.

breathe through the simulated contraction. It is a good idea if your partner varies the "contractions," sometimes going up and down regularly and giving you a rest in between, sometimes going up fast, down fast and then into the next one before you've had a chance to take your resting breath. It is also a good idea to change places once in a while, as this can give help your partner understand what you are trying to do and how to help you with your breathing if things get tough during labor.

CARING FOR YOUR BREASTS

By now your breasts may be leaking some colostrum. This is perfectly normal: colostrum will provide your baby with all the nutrients he needs before your breast milk comes in. These days it is not considered advisable to express the colostrum, but keep your breasts clean by washing them gently with soap and water. If you are worried about staining your clothes, start using breast pads. You will need them anyway, once the baby is born.

PERINEUM MASSAGE

Massaging your perineum may help to make it more supple and stretchy. This may help you avoid an episiotomy—a surgical cut to make the birth opening bigger. The perineal area softens anyway as you get closer to delivery, but massage may make it less likely to tear during the birth. Massage may also soften previous episiotomy scars. The best time to massage is after a warm bath. You can use vitamin E oil or Calendula ointment or a special perinatal massage oil.

PRACTICING POSITIONS FOR LABOR

During the later weeks of pregnancy you can also experiment with a variety of different positions you may find helpful once you go into labor.

■ In the early first stage you may feel happier walking about or standing up, supported by your partner. If you have low backache, you might want to kneel on all-fours or lean forward onto a chair or a heavy piece of furniture.

■ Once labor gets underway it may help if you already know what positions you feel comfortable with. You may find that during labor you want to change positions several times, so trying out as many as possible will give you a wide choice.

USEFUL POSITIONS TO TRY

Experiment with a range of different positions before you go into labor to find out which ones you feel most comfortable in. For example, you could try kneeling on the floor with your arms and head resting on a chair. This position may be useful as labor progresses and the contractions come harder and faster.

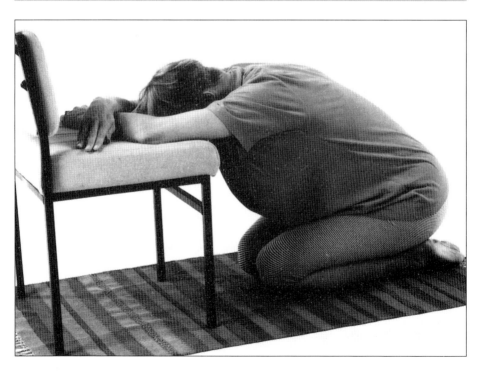

POSITIONS THAT EASE BACKACHE

Below: many women adopt this position of kneeling on all-fours during labor. This position is good for preventing or easing backache as it enables the uterus to fall forward.

Bottom: squatting down on your toes and leaning forward on to your hands for support can help take the weight off your back and helps you to work with gravity. This position needs practice.

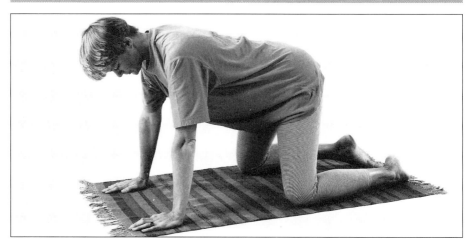

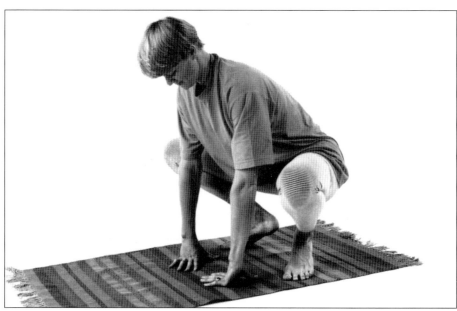

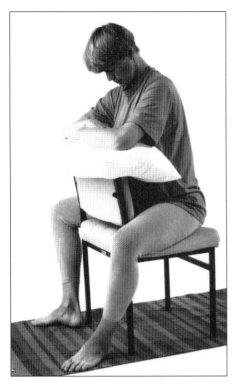

SUPPORTED POSITIONS FOR LABOR

Left: when you feel a contraction coming on, you can try sitting astride a chair the wrong way round.

Below left: put a pillow or cushion on the back of the chair and lean forward against it. Both these positions enable you to stay relatively upright and help speed up your labor.

Below: alternatively, you can kneel on the floor, using a chair for support, with your arms resting on the seat.

Note: all these positions can help you during labor and may even speed it up, as they work with gravity rather than against it. Rather than wait for the experience of labor, try practicing the positions in advance to discover which ones suit you best.

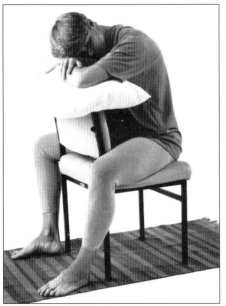

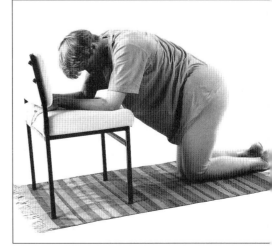

CHAPTER SIX

NATURAL BIRTH

Fairly early on in your pregnancy you need to start thinking about the kind of birth you would like to have. This gives you time to gather the information you will need to make informed choices about a range of issues, from where you would like to give birth, to what kind of pain relief, if any, you would like to use.

Once you have gathered this information you can use it to draw up a birth plan, which is a record of what you would like to happen during labor and birth. Write down what you want and keep a copy with you. You can use your birth plan to discuss things with your midwife and your doctor, so that they have a chance to get to know you better, understand your feelings, and recognize what your priorities are.

NATURAL BIRTH

Many women hope for a natural birth, with as little medical intervention as possible. Their aim is to rely on the support of a birth companion and midwives, to use self-help methods—including relaxation and breathing—to cope with pain, and to adopt the kind of positions that facilitate a straightforward labor and delivery.

MODERN TECHNOLOGY

Other women prefer to opt for maximum pain relief and a more medically managed labor, taking advantage of whatever modern technology is available.

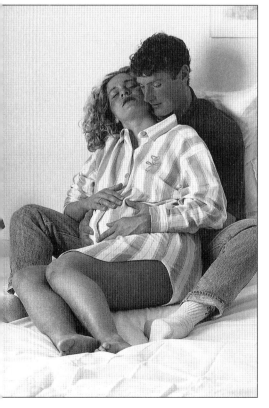

Left and opposite: you can use relaxation and breathing techniques to cope with pain. If your partner is with you, you can lean against him so that he can support and encourage you.

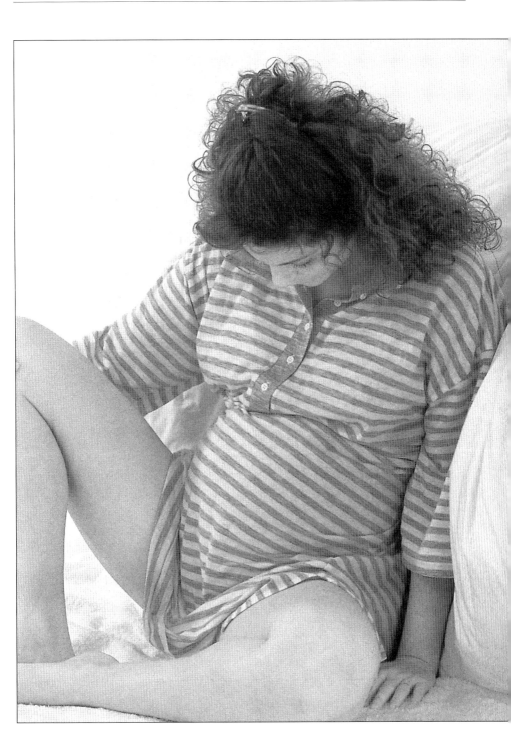

WHICH BIRTH?

Women who choose to manage naturally tend to report a high level of satisfaction with the experience. Without drugs you stay alert, and can take a more active role. You will be less likely to need medical intervention and more likely to be able to deliver your baby without assistance. Babies born without drugs in their system are more likely to be alert and responsive, and able to establish feeding without any problems.

That said, it is worth noting that many women plan one kind of birth and have another. Sometimes this is because labor did not go as expected. Sometimes it is because what they planned for—an epidural or a birthing pool, for instance—was not available at the time it was needed. And it is also worth knowing that if labor is particularly difficult, and the mother is under a great deal of stress, this can affect the baby's oxygen supply. Under those circumstances, accepting the offer of some kind of pain relief may be best for you and the baby.

Whatever happens on the day, the more you know about the kind of choices you have, the more flexible you can be, and the more you will feel in control. Even if you have planned for a natural birth, it is important not to approach the event as if it were some kind of examination which you will pass or fail. In the end, what matters is that you and your baby come through as safe and well as possible.

To a large extent, the choices you make about the kind of birth you would like will depend on where you live and what is available locally. Your obstetrician and your midwives should have information about different options in your area. Local hospitals should be able to give you information about the services they offer. You should also talk to some new mothers and local antenatal class teachers, to pick their brains about what goes on where. Remember, although health professionals will give you advice based on your medical history and any previous pregnancies, in the end the choices you make are yours. And if you opt for something to begin with, there is no reason why you can't change your mind later.

HOSPITAL BIRTH

Doctors often tell women that a hospital birth is much safer than having a baby at home. However, a U.K. review of the safety of home and hospital birth (*Where to be Born? The Debate and the Evidence*, published by the National Perinatal Epidemiology Unit in Oxford) concluded:

"The available evidence does not support claims that, for the baby, the iatrogenic (doctor-caused) risks of obstetric intervention outweigh the possible benefits.

Opposite: home or hospital delivery? The choice is yours, but health professionals will advise according to your medical history.

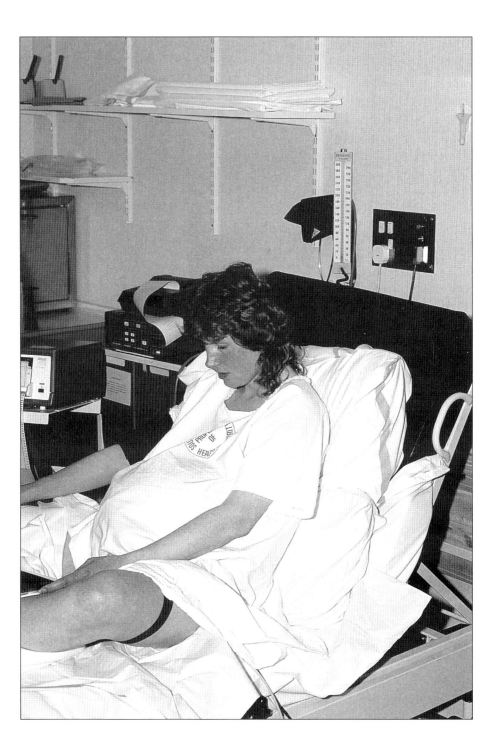

At the same time, there is no evidence to support the claim that the shift to hospital delivery is responsible for the decline in perinatal mortality in England and Wales, nor the claim that the safest policy is for women to be delivered in hospital."

Despite this, many women prefer the idea of a hospital delivery because they feel safer there or because they feel a home birth would not be appropriate in their particular circumstances. Many U.K. hospitals have now gone to some lengths to meet their patients' wishes in order to make maternity care more "woman-centered" and the U.K. government has even launched a campaign, which aims to give women a greater say in how their babies are born.

HOSPITAL BIRTHS

If you are considering a hospital birth, find out which hospitals you could go to and what goes on in each. Every hospital runs its maternity services in different ways. For instance, in some hospitals, midwives may work under the authority of obstetricians. In others, midwives may work in small teams, taking responsibility for the entire care of pregnant women, delivering their babies, and only referring them to doctors if they need specialist care. If a hospital talks about "team" care, you need to check out exactly what they mean by this statement. With true team midwifery you will probably see the same midwife every time you have an antenatal appointment, and she will most likely be the midwife who delivers you. Under a different system you may see different midwives at different times.

■ You should find out well in advance of labor, ideally in the early months of your pregnancy, exactly what facilities your chosen hospital can offer you. Ask about their routine procedures and whether they have an official policy on different aspects of labor, pain relief and birth. Don't wait until you actually go into labor to state your preferences and then discover that what you want is not possible. Talk to your midwife and obstetrician now and plan ahead.

■ Hospitals differ, too, in the kind of surroundings they offer women in labor. Some hospitals have delivery rooms decorated in a more homely style, with easy chairs, bean bags, or wedges so that women can move around and change position during labor. Some will be happy to put mattresses on the floor. Some may offer women a warm bath or shower, which can be soothing during the first stage of labor. Some may even have birthing pools available.

■ Routine procedures may vary from place to place, too. The practice of shaving off a woman's pubic hair has virtually disappeared as it is now known that it does not promote better hygiene and causes discomfort later on as the hair grows back. Some hospitals may still routinely recommend an enema or suppository to clear out your bowel although this is only really necessary if

CHECKLIST

When you go to the hospital for antenatal care, ask the staff the following questions to find out about the hospital's policies on birth and labor.

■ Am I likely to be delivered by a midwife I already know?

■ Will the same midwife stay with me throughout labor and delivery?

■ Who can be with me when I'm in labor—my partner, a friend, a relative, a complementary therapist?

■ Could I have more than one person with me?

■ Would my companion be allowed to stay throughout any examinations or procedures, including a Cesarean section if one was necessary?

■ Is there anywhere for my companion to get food and drink?

■ Will I be allowed to eat and drink during labor?

■ Will I be allowed to walk around in early labor—if so, where?

■ How will you monitor me and the baby—electronically or otherwise?

■ Is fetal blood sampling routine?

■ What pain relief is available—and is it available 24 hours a day?

■ Are your midwives encouraged to give positive support to women who want to avoid medical methods of pain relief?

■ Do you have cushions and wedges—can I bring my own?

■ Are there floor mats or bean bags if I don't feel able to get up on a bed?

■ Do you have a birthing bed or a birthing pool—how would I arrange to use it?

■ Do any of the obstetricians have a policy of speeding up labor artificially if it seems to be going slowly?

■ If so, what methods are usually used—and are women usually electronically monitored during labor?

■ Under what circumstances would you induce labor—and how?

■ How long do most women take in the second, pushing stage?

■ What is the most common position for women to give birth in? What other positions are used?

■ Are midwives and obstetricians happy to deliver me in whatever position I find comfortable?

■ Is there an official hospital policy on episiotomies and how many women have them?

■ Can midwives do stitching—if not, will I be stitched by a trained doctor?

■ How is the baby usually delivered?

■ Can cord cutting be delayed and pitocin be avoided unless problems develop?

■ Will I be able to suckle my baby after delivery?

■ Are the babies in a nursery or by their mothers' beds?

■ Who helps with breastfeeding and are mothers encouraged to feed on demand?

■ What services are there for sick babies?

■ What is the normal length of stay for most mothers?

■ Are there any rules about visitors and visiting hours?

you are constipated, which could impede the delivery.

■ In some places you may be discouraged from eating or taking more than sips of water during labor. In fact, restricting food and drink during labor may lead to dehydration and ketosis, both of which are potentially hazardous. There is no guarantee that fasting will mean you have an empty stomach if you need a general anesthetic in an emergency so check with your midwife. It is better to eat and drink if you feel like it although it is probably best to stick to easily digestible, low-fat foods. You may want to sip water or fruit juice, nibble some toast or plain cookies or have some fruit.

MAKE A LIST

One way of finding out what goes on in a hospital is to draw up a list of questions. Only you will know which aspects of your care are most important to you, but it will help you decide what you might need to ask (see page 75).

You can learn quite a lot about the underlying ethos of a particular hospital from the way in which the replies to your questions are given. There is a world of difference between a hospital where a midwife says, "Most women give birth in a sitting position, propped up by extra pillows. But some find it more comfortable kneeling or squatting," and one where she says, "Most women give birth in a sitting position, propped up by extra pillows. But some seem to think they'll get on better if they kneel or squat."

KNEELING POSITIONS

A variety of different kneeling positions can be helpful during the transition stage of labor. You might like to try some of the positions illustrated here. You could try practicing them beforehand in readiness for the birth.

Below: some women find that squatting is a good position. It needs practice and can be tiring if you are unaccustomed to it. However, it does enable you to stay upright so that gravity works with you, not against you. Thus, in theory, your baby's head can press down, the cervix dilates faster and the labor should be shorter.

Opposite above: you may feel more comfortable in a kneeling position with your head, shoulders and arms supported by some cushions or pillows.

Opposite below: an alternative kneeling position is just to kneel on the floor with your bottom up in the air. Lean forward with your elbows bent until your lower arms and head are resting on the floor.

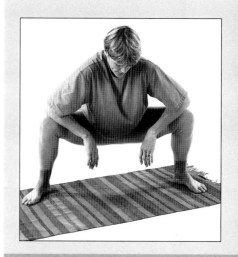

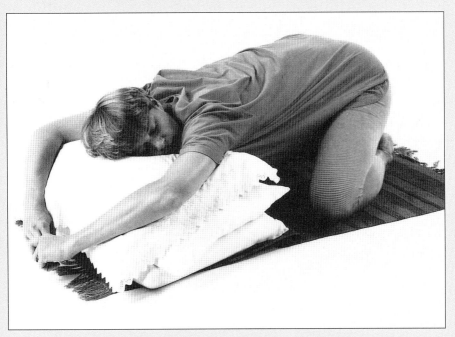

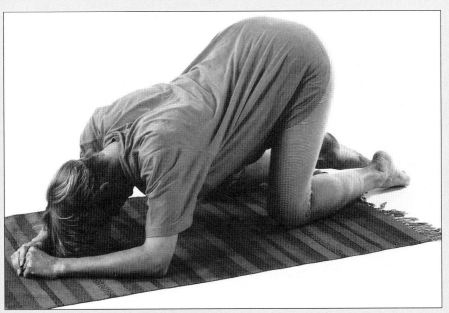

CHOICES IN LABOR AND CHILDBIRTH

ACTIVE MANAGEMENT OF LABOR

Women are less likely these days to be started off in labor artificially unless there are clear medical indications that either the mother or baby will be at risk if the pregnancy continues as it is. Labor can be induced in a number of ways: a prostaglandin pessary may be put in your vagina to ripen your cervix, your waters may be broken (this is known as ARM—artificial rupture of the membranes) or you may be put on a drip containing an oxytocic drug.

Even if your labor starts naturally, doctors may suggest speeding things up if it seems to be progressing slowly. This is known as active management of labor.

Induction is not always successful in starting labor. If it is tried and fails you will probably need a Cesarean—which is why doctors need to feel very sure that an induction is necessary before they start taking matters into their own hands.

If it is possible, natural alternatives may be worth trying before you get to this point. Some women say that having sex triggered off labor: semen contains prostaglandin. Another suggestion is to try rubbing your nipples for at least 15 minutes at a time which may stimulate your natural production of oxytocin.

SPEEDING UP LABOR NATURALLY

The simplest way to try to speed up labor is to keep your body upright and move

> ### COMPLEMENTARY MEDICINE
>
> Some complementary therapies may prove helpful in the management of labor.
> - Cranial osteopathy and reflexology may help in labor.
> - Homeopaths suggest caulophyllum, which may also help speed up labor.
> - There are herbal remedies, such as goldenseal, for encouraging contractions to become stronger and more regular.

around. When you change position, you alter the relationship between gravity, the contractions, your baby, and the pelvis, and this may enhance the progress of labor and reduce pain.

Trials have shown that women who asked to stand, walk, or sit upright had on average shorter labors than women who asked to stay lying down. The evidence also suggests that lying down means that the uterus works less effectively, so women tend to need more pain relief and drugs to speed things up.

> ### THREE STAGES OF LABOR
>
> There are three stages to labor.
> - During stage one, the cervix dilates.
> - In stage two, the baby is pushed down the vagina and born.
> - In stage three, the placenta comes away and is delivered.

THE BIRTH

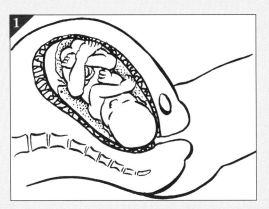

1 The cervix is almost completely dilated here toward the end of the first stage of labor, although the bag of fluid is still intact. By the time the cervix has dilated to four inches, you will get the urge to bear down and push your baby out through the birth canal.

2 You have to work hard to push your baby out in the second stage of labor. Your baby's head will eventually appear in the opening to the birth canal, with the face turned toward your back.

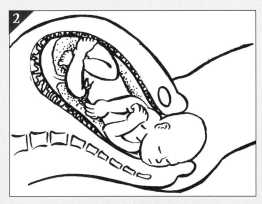

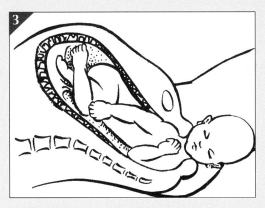

3 The baby's head will then emerge and as he slides out through the perineum, you can push out the shoulders. You will feel your baby slithering out of you and will be able to hold him in your arms at last. However, the labor is not yet over, and during the third and final stage, the placenta comes away and is delivered.

LABOR

A t the start of labor, contractions help to soften the cervix which then gradually opens. Sometimes the softening process can go on for a long time before the cervix is about one inch open and you have reached what midwives call established labor. Eventually the cervix opens to about four inches. It is then described as being fully dilated, and this means the cervix is now wide enough to let the baby out.

Once labor is established you will be checked regularly to see how you are progressing. Towards the end of the first

Below: midwives can check your baby's heartbeat during your labor without using electronic monitoring.

stage you may feel you want to push, but before you start you should be checked by the midwife to ensure your cervix is fully dilated and the baby's head can be seen.

MONITORING YOUR BABY'S HEARTBEAT

Throughout labor your baby's heartbeat will be checked. If there are any changes in the rhythm this could be an indication that the baby is in difficulties. This can be confirmed by testing the baby's blood and may mean that a Cesarean or a forceps delivery is needed to deliver the baby quickly.

■ There are different ways of monitoring fetal heartbeat. The midwife or obstetrician can listen by holding a portable, hand-held

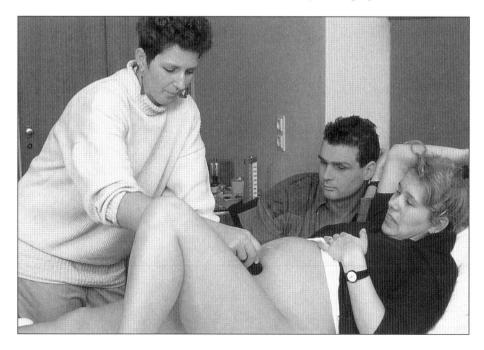

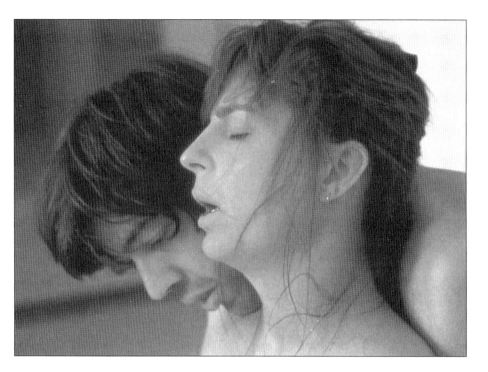

ultrasound detector or doppler, which is held against your stomach and amplifies the baby's heartbeat.

■ Many hospitals use electronic monitors, which can give continuous ultrasound monitoring throughout a woman's labor. These monitors transmit information to a machine which bleeps and makes a print out. The monitor is either held against your stomach by a belt or connected to the baby's scalp by a tiny metal clip on a lead, put on during a vaginal examination. In some hospitals the scalp monitor transmits information via radio waves to a remote monitor so no wires connecting you to the machine are necessary.

■ Since it is an advantage in labor to be able to adopt upright positions and move

Above: your partner can offer practical and emotional support throughout labor.

around as you feel like it, you may prefer to be monitored by a doppler. This won't restrict your movements at all and you will be able to move around if you so wish. Electronic monitoring is usually restrictive and studies have shown little difference in the effectiveness of continuous electronic monitoring and intermittent monitoring by a midwife.

■ That said, some hospital obstetricians use electronic monitoring routinely and most prefer to rely on it if labor has been going on for a long time, if you have been given drugs to induce or accelerate labor, or if you are having an epidural.

■ Of course, if there is a particular reason to be worried about the baby, then electronic monitoring can be reassuring both for you and the staff. The trouble is that inaccurate readings or careless interpretation of the data can lead to emergency intervention when it is not actually necessary. Some physicians may choose to perform a fetal blood sampling as a back-up measure before emergency action is taken.

Walking around and being mobile in the early stages of your labor, helps to make it progress faster. Check in advance with the hospital staff whether you will be able to walk around. Unless there is some cause for concern, it should not be necessary for you to be confined to bed to be monitored. Although you are mobile, the nursing staff can still take your temperature, check your blood pressure and check the baby's heartbeat on a regular basis throughout the early stages of labor.

PAIN RELIEF IN LABOR

If you are hoping for a natural birth, you will probably want to manage your labor without the aid of any drugs. Most physicians and midwives agree that it is best to keep the use of pain-relieving drugs to a minimum if possible. However, these drugs do have their uses, and if you have a difficult or complicated labor, you may need to use them. Therefore it will help you to know what kinds of pain relief may be offered to you, and the effect that they

could have on both you and your baby.

Pain relief is now very sophisticated and need not involve altering your state of consciousness. Ask your physician what forms of pain relief will be available should you need them, and get him/her to explain their effects on you and your baby. Nubane is the most commonly used type of pain relief. However, it is possible that you may need an epidural, so you should find out about this too.

If your physician or midwife decides that some form of pain relief is necessary when you go into labor, make sure that you understand and approve of what they propose giving you. If your partner is with you, he can help to ask the right questions so that the procedures can be explained.

A labor and delivery department in a big hospital can be quite intimidating and it is only natural to have some fears about the birth and how painful it will be. However, sometimes the anticipation of pain can make the experience more painful than it might otherwise have been. But don't worry—you can have pain relief if you need it. In fact, a small amount of the right sort of pain relief may be beneficial for you and the way in which your labor progresses.

The exercises, positions for labor and breathing exercises that you practiced at antenatal classes will have helped to prepare you for the experience of labor so that you are better able to cope with it, but even these skills and your endurance may not be enough when the time comes. You

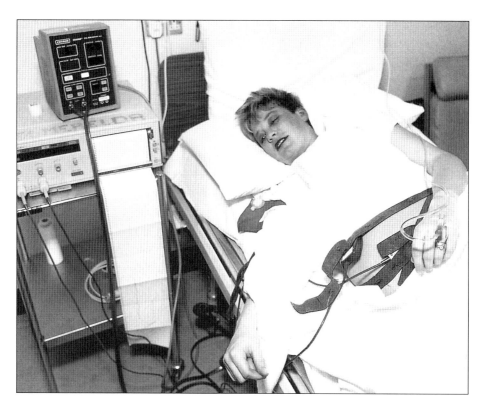

should not regard yourself as a failure if you planned for a natural birth but end up taking some pain-relieving drugs. Things can't always go the way we plan and accepting pain relief if you feel exhausted, or unable to cope with the pain, or if there is an unforeseen complication in your labor, is perfectly understandable and the sensible thing to do in the circumstances. Just be flexible when the moment arrives and do what seems best.

Above: during the early stages of labor, sophisticated equipment is often used for fetal monitoring. However, this may interfere with your ability to walk around.

■ EPIDURAL

This is an anesthetic to numb the nerves which carry pain messages to the brain. After a local anesthetic in your back you lie

on your side or sit up while a needle is inserted into a space between the bones in your spine. A thin tube is then attached and the needle withdrawn. Anesthetic can then be dripped through the tube into the epidural space in your back so that you become numb below the waist. A drip will be attached to your hand and if you can't feel your bladder, a catheter will be inserted. The whole procedure takes about 20 minutes and, because it can only be done by a trained anesthetist, it may not be available in every hospital or at all times.

An epidural is the most effective form of pain relief and may mean a completely pain-free labor. If you need a Cesarean together with a spinal anaesthetic, it is the safest form of anesthetic for mother and baby and means you are awake and alert when your baby is born.

Some women are offered an epidural if their labor is long and particularly painful. In those circumstances, having

Below: the support of a partner or a close companion can be the best pain relief of all during your labor.

an epidural may help because you are likely to feel less tired afterwards. On the other hand, as you will not be able to feel the contractions you will have to be electronically monitored—and the drip, the anesthetic, and the monitor will restrict your movements. This, in itself may slow things down and may result in the doctor suggesting drugs to speed things up. Most hospitals find that women who have an epidural are more likely to end up needing a forceps or Cesarean delivery. This may be because the aesthetic reduces the urge to push. If you can't feel your contractions then you may have to be told when to push rather than following your natural

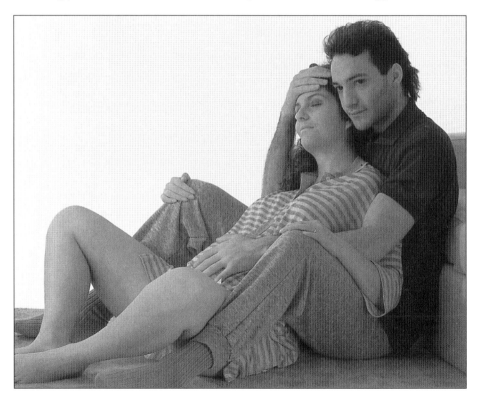

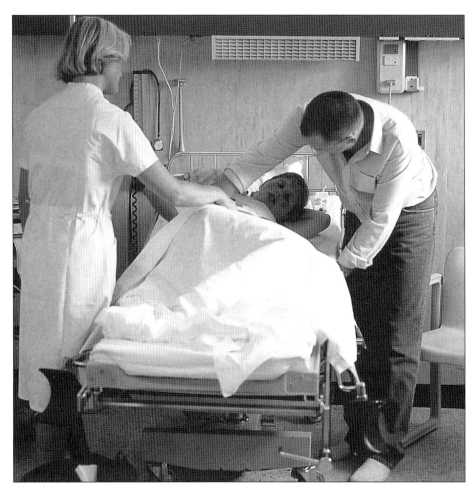

instincts. That's why some anesthetists allow the effects of the anesthetic to wear off in the second stage of labor. However, it is worth noting that the force of late labor pains can then come as a shock to the woman concerned.

Some women who have been given an epidural get backache or a temporary loss of sensation in their legs afterwards. A few women suffer from headaches and severe nausea which may last for several days.

Above: if the labor is long and seems never-ending, your partner can be wonderfully reassuring and supportive. He can help you breathe through the contractions.

Other women have difficulty urinating after the delivery. There is also the extremely remote risk of an accident when putting the tube in or administering the anesthetic. In a few rare cases, this has led to paralysis or death.

SELF-HELP

Having the right kind of support is one of the most effective pain relievers. That is why it helps if you go into labor with your partner or a companion who knows you well and understands what you are trying to do. A companion can give you comfort and moral support. They can keep you company and help you pass the time in the early stages. They can remind you to empty your bladder every hour or so—a full bladder can hold up labor and make it feel more painful. They can wipe your face, give you sips of water, massage you, help you move about or change position. They can remind you about the breathing and relaxation techniques you have learned, breathing with you if that helps. They can support your decisions—about monitoring or pain relief—and act as a go-between and interpreter, so that the midwives and doctors are clear about what you need and vice versa. And as your baby is being born they can tell you what is happening.

A supportive companion or midwife can also help you deal with pain by focusing on its purpose and your progress, rather than the pain itself. Just as athletes focus on a goal—the end of the race—rather than their aching muscles, so you may need to be reminded that you are doing really well, that each contraction is one less to go, one step nearer the birth of your baby.

RELAXATION IN LABOR

Some studies suggest that music has the capacity to reduce pain. You may like to

---

HELP IN LABOR

What else might help? Simple measures, such as putting a hot water bottle on your back or stomach, or having a warm bath are worth a try. You might find cold rather than warmth helps; try using freezellas instead. It helps if you feel as comfortable as possible between contractions. A water spray will help keep you cool and freshen you up. A pair of socks will keep your feet warm. A lip balm will keep your lips moist.

---

use headphones during labor. Listening to music may help block out distractions and encourage relaxation or visualization.

You could imagine a a range of mountains, with trees on the lower slopes and snow on the very top of the highest ones. As a contraction builds, imagine yourself beginning to lift yourself up the side of the first mountain. Then, as the force builds, you go higher and higher, changing up through your breathing levels as you go. As the contraction fades you float down the other side. When the contractions are at their strongest, picture the highest mountains of all and see yourself lifting yourself up and up, right over the topmost peak.

In between contractions when you want to relax, you could get in a comfortable position and close your eyes. Listen to the natural flow of your breathing and then start to imagine yourself walking along a beach. The sand is warm, soft, and golden. The water is clear and blue, lapping at your feet. Palm trees wave softly in the gentle breeze along the fringes of the beach. You lie down at the water's edge, letting the little waves wash gently over you. With each wave you feel your tension being washed away. You feel invigorated. Now let the image fade and start to become aware of your surroundings. Take a deep breath and open your eyes.

COMPLEMENTARY MEDICINE

■ Acupuncture

Acupuncture can reduce nausea, relieve pain, and speed up a slow labor, but you must arrange to have your therapist with you.

■ Homeopathy

If you would like to use homeopathic remedies, you should consult a practitioner well in advance of your labor, as everyone is different and remedies are prescribed on an individual basis. However, you could take a homeopathic first aid kit with you. Caulophyllum may make contractions more effective; Kali Phos may help if you are becoming exhausted with a long labor; Gelsemium is for trembling and weakness; Pulsatilla if you are weepy and indecisive and need comfort; Aconite may reduce anxiety.

■ Herbal medicine

Herbal remedies include Raspberry leaf tea, sipped or sucked as ice cubes, or Bach Rescue Remedy to ward off exhaustion. An infusion of Mugwort may also help establish strong, regular contractions.

■ Massage

Massage can also be used to relieve pain, although some women find they cannot bear to be touched during labor. Getting your partner to massage your neck and shoulders with their thumbs can help ease tension. Using the heel of the hand against the base of the spine and rubbing in a circular motion can also be good for relieving backache. Aromatherapists suggest using Clary Sage in the massage oil.

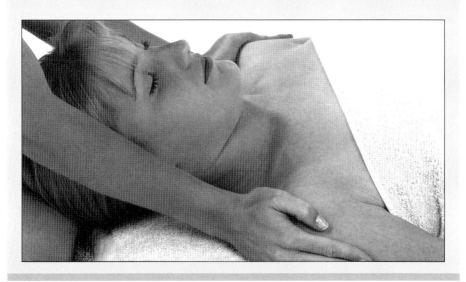

POSITIONS FOR LABOR

During the first stage of labor you need to feel free to walk around or adopt a comfortable position.

■ You may want to sit astride a chair. If you put a cushion over the back and lean

Below: sitting astride a chair helps your body work with gravity.

forward against it, your body will be supported, yet vertical, and your pelvis open. Your partner can massage your back.

■ Another position you might find useful is supported kneeling. You kneel down with your toes together and your knees apart and then lean forward over some cushions or a piece of furniture.

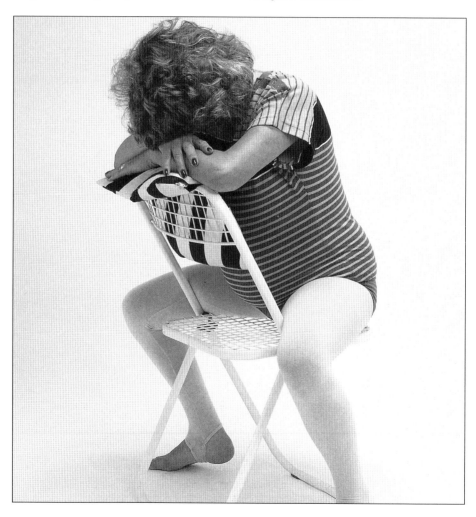

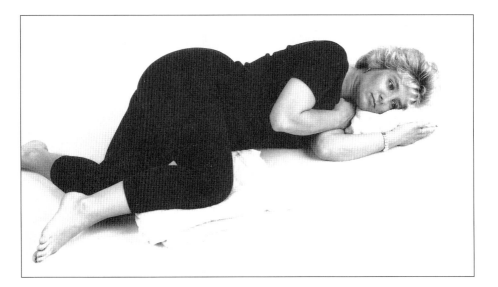

■ You might want to stay upright, on your feet, leaning forward against a wall or your partner for support. Upright positions like this make the most of the forces of gravity to stimulate contractions and help the progress of labor.

■ Squatting can help, too, but not all women come from cultures where squatting is as natural as sitting. Your partner may be able to support you if he kneels down facing you so that you can clasp your hands round his neck.

■ Many women like to circle or rock their hips. Kneeling on all-fours makes this easy. If the contractions become very powerful you can put your head down to the floor, leaving your bottom in the air, which can help to slow things up, allowing you to stay in control.

■ At some point you may feel like lying down, especially if labor has been going on for a while and you are getting tired. Don't

Above: if labor is prolonged and you are getting tired, lie down on your side.

lie on your back as this can affect the flow of blood to your womb. Try lying on your side, with your bump propped up by some pillows or cushions.

POSITIONS IN TRANSITION

At the end of the first stage you will go into transition. This is the time when you may find it hardest to cope. The contractions may feel more painful, you may be weepy or irritable, shaking, or shivering. You may also feel the urge to push but it is important to wait until the midwife has checked that your cervix is fully dilated. You may find that panting or special transitional breathing (see page 66) helps. Another trick is to kneel on all-fours, with your head down and your bottom up. This reduces the pressure of the baby's head on your cervix.

POSITIONS IN THE SECOND STAGE

In the second stage of labor, which leads to the birth of your baby, you need to find a position which is comfortable and efficient. Lying flat on your back is the worst position of all. Many women are encouraged to give birth lying propped up against cushions or a wedge. This is not ideal, either. As your baby's head comes through your pelvis, your coccyx (tailbone) should flip out of the way. But if you are sitting on your bottom, your coccyx will be squashed.

■ If you feel comfortable about squatting you could try a supported squat—although if you think this is what you will want to do, it is probably better to have practiced it before labor begins. Your partner kneels down while you squat in front, your back to his chest. You lift your arms so he can pass his arms underneath, then clasp them in front of your chest to hold you up. Then you lean back against him with your knees wide apart.

Other positions women find helpful in the second stage are kneeling ones. You can either kneel on all-fours or adopt a supported kneeling position

THE PLACENTA

This cross-section through the placenta shows the maternal arteries and veins and the umbilical cord. Your blood filters through the intervillous spaces. Nutrients can slip through and be transferred to the baby. In the same way, waste products can be transferred to the mother. Do remember that other harmful substances can also percolate through this strainer, including drugs and toxic chemicals.

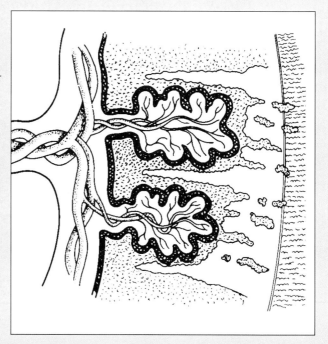

with the help of your partner.

■ Unless your baby is in distress there is no reason why you should be encouraged or directed to make vigorous pushing efforts. Recent evidence suggests that making short pushing efforts and panting or breathing gently in between allows the tissues time to relax and stretch under pressure.

■ This may also help you avoid an episiotomy—a cut in the perineum. Episiotomy may be necessary if forceps have to be used. However, sometimes women are offered one on the grounds that a cut heals better than a tear.

DELIVERY OF THE PLACENTA

After your baby is born you still have to deliver the placenta. In most cases this can happen without any medical intervention, but in modern hospitals a number of medical techniques are routinely employed. An injection of a drug called pitocin is usually given in your thigh as the baby is being delivered. This makes the womb contract.

To avoid trapping the placenta, the baby's cord is cut and clamped at once. Then the midwife may pull gently on your end of it to speed up the delivery of the placenta.

If you want things to take their natural course (unless problems develop during or after delivery) you should have discussed this with your midwife in advance and made sure there is a note of this on your birth plan. If you don't want a routine injection of pitocin, the cord should not be cut until the placenta is delivered.

WATER BIRTHS

A growing number of women are interested in the idea of using water pools for labor and/or birth. Being immersed in water can help make labor shorter, easier and less painful and may help give the baby a gentle entry into the world.

Some hospitals have their own pools. Others allow you to hire one of your own which can be set up for you to use. These are supplied with disposable liners, hosepipes to help you fill the pool, a floating thermometer so you can monitor the pool temperature, and a pumping system to empty the water out again. The average cost of hiring a pool will vary, so check this out first. For more information on water births, ask your midwife or obstetrician.

Bleeding after the birth—post partum hemorrhage—used to be a real danger and many doctors think the routine use of pitocin has made childbirth much safer. However, if you do start to bleed heavily, the bleeding can be stopped by an intravenous injection of ergometrine, which will contract the womb in seconds. This is worth knowing if someone wants to give you pitocin and you think there is no reason to do so.

One natural way of encouraging the uterus to contract is to put your baby to your breast. Herbal remedies can also be useful and include Southernwood, Wormwood, Mugwort, Cloves, Goldenseal, Rue, Nutmeg, and Penny Royal.

HOME BIRTHS

Many experienced childbirth campaigners believe that the best way to have the kind of birth you want is to have a home birth. Having a baby at home can be more private and special. There will be no question of having to fit into a hospital routine and you are less likely to be pressured into making use of whatever medical and technological help is available, whether you or your baby need it or not.

You are more likely to get to know the midwife who delivers you, and she will be in tune with your priorities and wishes. At home you may feel more relaxed and better able to cope in familiar surroundings. However, getting a home birth may not be as easy as it should be. Some doctors and midwives believe that home births are not as safe as hospital births. In fact, there is no statistical evidence to show that in a straightforward pregnancy, it is less safe for a woman to have a baby at home than in a hospital.

In any case, it is the right of every woman to have a home birth if that is what she wishes. Any woman who wants to have her baby at home should talk it through with her obstetrician and midwife before making a decision. Having a home birth is not dependent on their approval, although obviously it would be sensible for a woman to listen to any professional advice before making up her mind what is best for herself and her baby.

Women who want a home birth should get a doctor to cover for the midwife. Of course, if you know your obstetrician is interested in doing home births, you can approach them and ask if they would be prepared to provide cover. If not, you can register with another obstetrician who is prepared to take on this task and attend you at home.

It is also possible to find an experienced midwife, who practices independently, who will take you on. However, this can be expensive and she may have access to fewer facilities in the case of an emergency. Before you decide to go ahead with plans for a home birth it is a good idea to arm yourself with as much information as possible and consider all the possibilities.

Opposite: giving birth to your baby at home in familiar surroundings can be very comforting and rewarding for both you and your partner.

RECOVERING NATURALLY

You can also use natural remedies to help you recover from the labor and the birth.
- Massaging a few drops of diluted Lavender oil into your temples may perk you up if you are feeling exhausted.
- Arnica helps heal bruising, while Calendula can help with soreness if you have had a tear or an episiotomy.
- Once the wound has healed you could try massaging the scar with some diluted Comfrey essential oil.

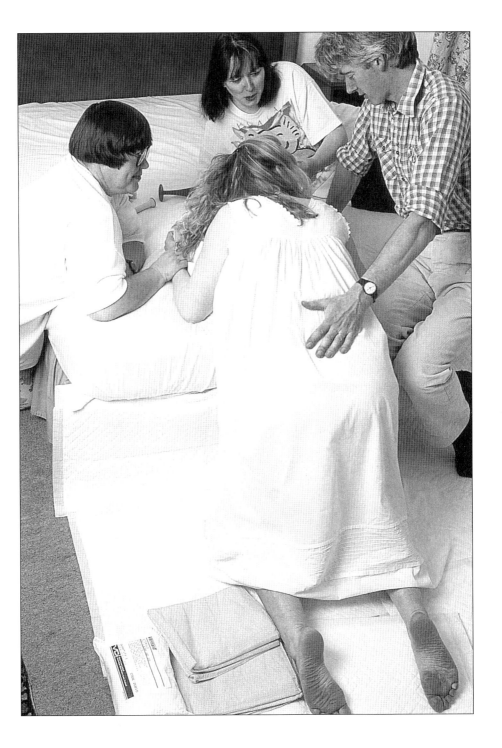

CHAPTER SEVEN

COMPLEMENTARY MEDICINE

Complementary medicine can be useful during pregnancy and labor; it provides a more natural non-invasive approach to pregnancy than does orthodox medicine.

Below: meditation and yoga are both relaxing forms of complementary medicine which will help reduce stress and calm your mind in readiness for birth.

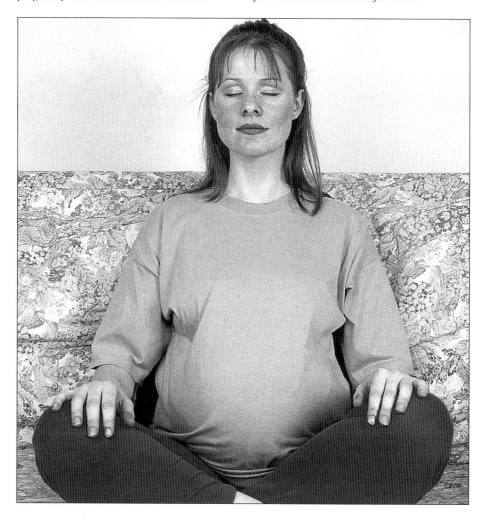

Only go to a qualified practitioner, and discuss it with your doctor. Complementary medicine should complement, not replace, conventional antenatal care.

ACUPUNCTURE

■ **What is it?**
Fine needles are inserted into the skin and left there for about 20 minutes. These stimulate points along energy lines known as meridians to redress the balance of the body.

■ **How can it help in pregnancy?**
It can be used to treat most common problems including sickness and physical aches and pains. It may encourage breech babies to turn naturally and can be used to stimulate the onset of labor. It may also be used as a method of pain relief during labor.

Caution: care must be taken, particularly in the early stages of pregnancy, not to stimulate certain points on each meridian, such as those that might stimulate the uterus.

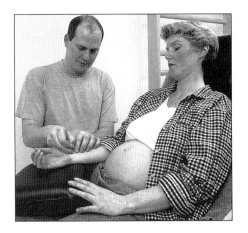

Above: acupuncture can be used to treat many minor complaints of pregnancy.

physical well-being by improving a person's posture and balance.

■ How can it help in pregnancy? It can help you adapt the way you move as you change shape, so avoiding backache. It can also be used to prepare for labor and birth by teaching you ways to release tension.

ACUPRESSURE

■ **What is it?**
It works in a similar way to acupuncture except that the points are stimulated by pressure, usually the therapist's fingertips.

■ **How can it help in pregnancy?**
It can relieve sickness and headaches as well as aches and pains. As with acupuncture, certain pressure points should be avoided during pregnancy.

ALEXANDER TECHNIQUE

■ **What is it?**
A method of enhancing mental and

AROMATHERAPY

■ **What is it?**
The use of essential oils, distilled from various plants, fruits, and herbs. The diluted oils are often used in a therapeutic massage. They can also be inhaled or added to compresses or baths.

■ **How can it help in pregnancy?**
It aids relaxation and may alleviate a range of minor problems from back pain to fluid retention.

Caution: some oils can be harmful. Those to avoid during pregnancy include Origanum, Sage, Thyme, Savoury,

Wintergreen, Black Pepper, Basil, Clove, Hyssop, Marjoram, Myrrh, Camphor, Cedarwood, Juniper, and Pennyroyal. Others may cause blotching if your skin is exposed to sunlight: these include Bergamot, Fennel, Grapefruit, Lemon, Lime, Mandarin, Orange, and Tangerine. Essential oils should always be diluted before use.

AUTOGENIC TRAINING

■ What is it?

A carefully designed sequence of mental exercises which allows the mind to calm itself by switching off the body's stress response. The standard exercise involves taking the focus inward and using mental repetition of a sequence of phrases relating to the body in its relaxed state.

■ How can it help in pregnancy?

Regular practice of the autogenic standard exercise, if started early in pregnancy, can prevent or alleviate some of problems such as nausea or insomnia. Autogenic training can be effective in the first stage of labor, helping women to cope with contractions without analgesics.

BACH FLOWER REMEDIES

■ What are they?

They aim to cure the emotional disharmony and instability which cause disease by using the subtle energy given off by plants.

■ How can they help in pregnancy?

They can help combat fatigue and lack of

Below: aromatherapy massage can be very relaxing and therapeutic during your pregnancy.

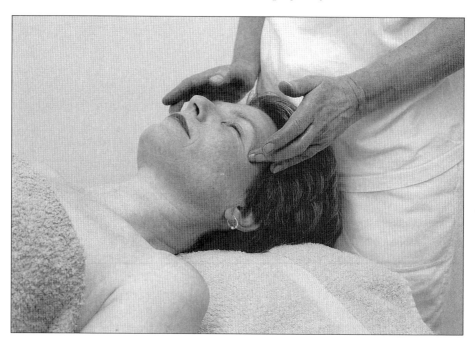

confidence. Rescue Remedy may be of help during labor.

CHIROPRACTIC

■ **What is it?**

Manual treatment of musculo-skeletal aches and pains.

■ **How can it help in pregnancy?**

Can help relieve back pain.

COLOR THERAPY

■ **What is it?**

The use of color to restore physical health and well-being. Therapists may use colored light or suggest which color clothes you should wear or foods you should eat. You may also be taught to visualize colors.

■ **How can it help in pregnancy?**

It may help with relaxation or insomnia.

COLOR BREATHING EXERCISE

Try the following exercise. Lie down comfortably with your spine relaxed, breathing naturally. Either breathe through the whole spectrum of colors suggested below, or choose a particular color for its specific qualities. Just relax and concentrate on visualizing your chosen color. As you practice this simple technique and become more adept at it, you should start to feel more relaxed and at peace.

Red	Base	Breathe in red for vitality. Breathe out turquoise.
Orange	Sacral	Breathe in orange for joy. Breathe out blue.
Yellow	Solar Plexus	Breathe in yellow for increased objectivity and intellectual powers. Breathe out violet.
Green	Heart	Breathe in green to cleanse and balance. Breathe out magenta.
Turquoise	Thymus	Breathe in turquoise to strengthen the immune system. Breathe out red.
Blue	Throat	Breathe in blue for relaxation. Breathe out orange.
Violet	Brow	Breathe in violet to increase self-respect, to connect with feelings of dignity and beauty. Breathe out yellow.
Magenta	Crown	Breathe in magenta to release obsessional images and thoughts. Breathe out green.

CRANIAL OSTEOPATHY

■ What is it?

Treatment by a qualified osteopath who works on your skull to restore the balance in your body via the fluid and membranes of your brain and spinal cord.

■ How can it help in pregnancy?

Treatment may release any compression in the pelvis so it can stretch fully during the process of birth.

HOMEOPATHY

■ What is it?

A system of medicine based upon the principle of treating like with like. That means the medication chosen for a particular patient would, if given in large quantities, produce the symptoms they are complaining of. In preparing the medicines, extracts of the plant or other material are made and then repeatedly diluted a hundredfold.

■ How can it help in pregnancy?

It can be used to treat nausea, fatigue, heartburn, insomnia, edema, piles, and skin complaints. Remedies may also be used to encourage the natural progression of labor. **Caution:** homeopathic medicines can be a safe alternative to drugs, but during pregnancy it is advisable to seek qualified advice from a qualified homeopath before embarking on any treatment.

HERBAL MEDICINE

■ What is it?

The use of herbs to relieve symptoms and improve general health.

■ How can it help in pregnancy?

Herbal preparations may be useful to promote sleep or relaxation. They may also alleviate problems such as sickness, piles, constipation, cramp, or varicose veins.
Caution: although herbs have been used for centuries, they can have powerful effects. Always read the label or accompanying leaflet carefully to make sure a preparation is safe to take or use during pregnancy and if you are in any doubt, seek qualified advice. Some herbs should be avoided in pregnancy: these include Aloe Vera, Autumn Crocus, Barberry, Broom, Juniper, Penny Royal, Poke Root, Parsley, Tansy, Thuja, Wormwood, Feverfew, and Saafras. Goldenseal should not be taken during pregnancy although it can be useful for stimulating contractions during labor.

NATUROPATHY

■ What is it?

Practitioners believe the body has the power to cure itself due to its inner life-force and natural instinctual wisdom. The aim of therapy is to stimulate the body's natural healing power and encourage it to retain its natural harmony and balance.

■ How can it help in pregnancy?

Naturopaths can advise you how to change your lifestyle and will promote a healthy, natural diet to maximize your well-being and that of your baby during pregnancy.

Opposite: as the birth of your baby approaches you can relax, knowing that you are both prepared for the birth.

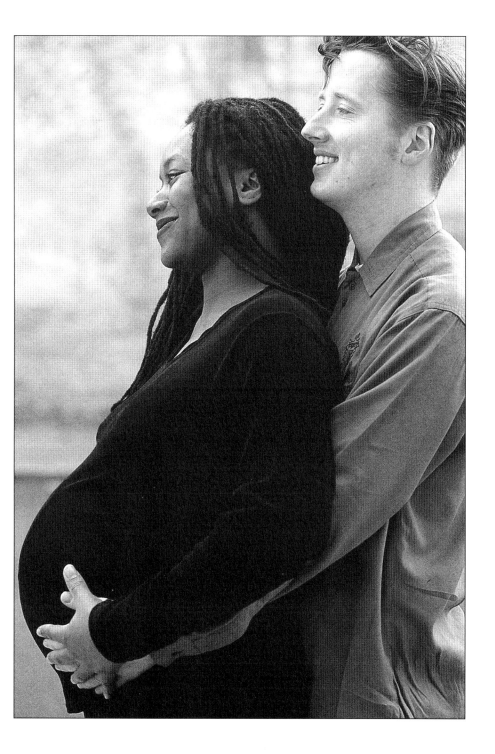

OSTEOPATHY

■ What is it?

Manipulation of the spine and other joints and massage of soft tissue to maintain or restore good health.

■ How can it help in pregnancy?

It can relieve backache and help to promote good posture. Manipulation of the joints may keep the body mobile and healthy at a time when there is extra strain on the back, hips, and knees due to the weight of the baby and the softening effect on the joints of pregnancy hormones.

REFLEXOLOGY

■ What is it?

Pressure applied to different parts of the feet which correspond to every organ and function of the body. The stimulation opens up energy channels in the body, thereby encouraging it to repair itself.

■ How can it help in pregnancy?

It can help reduce stress and anxiety and is also used to treat fatigue, sickness, swollen ankles, and constipation.

YOGA

■ What is it?

An Indian tradition based on stretching exercises (known as postures or *asanas*) combined with controlled breathing and relaxation to bring the mind and body into harmony. In Iyenga yoga there is a group of asanas specifically tailored to release stress, physically and mentally.

■ How can it help in pregnancy?

Yoga can help physically and mentally. The exercises can help increase strength and suppleness as well as teaching you how to relax and breathe more effectively.

Below: consider a range of complementary medicine such as reflexology or yoga (opposite) to make your experience of pregnancy and childbirth as natural as possible. Always seek expert advice.

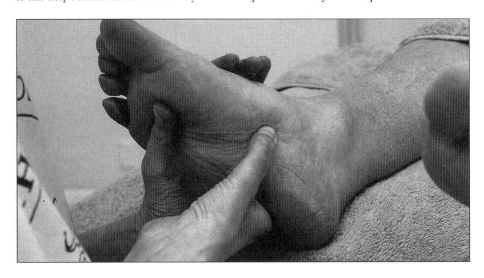

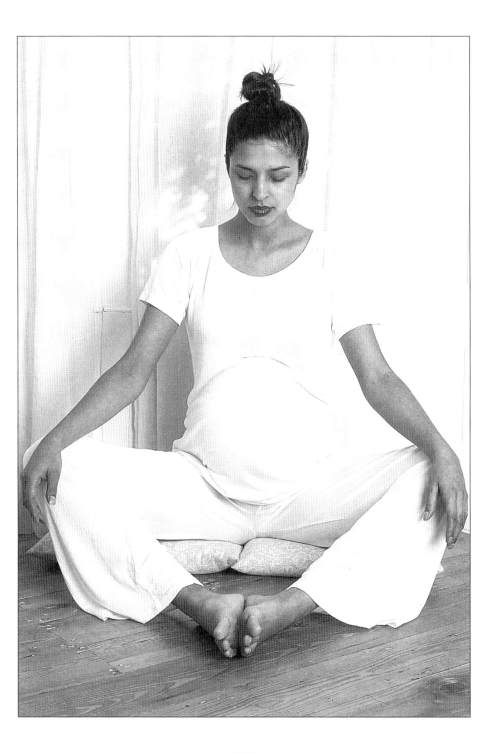

PROGRESS IN PREGNANCY

PRECONCEPTION

Review your diet and lifestyle. Have a preconception health check. Introduce regular exercise if you are not very active. Make sure you are immune to rubella—or get vaccinated against it. If you smoke, try to stop, cut down on alcohol, and eat a balanced diet. Take folic acid supplements. Avoid environmental hazards. Find ways to relax and reduce stress.

CONCEPTION

Pregnancy is dated from the first day of your last period. So the week of conception becomes week three of a forty-week pregnancy.

0—8 WEEKS

■ By week four—the date when your period should have started—the fertilized egg will have embedded in the uterine lining. It is nourished by the blood vessels there. You can use a urine sample to do a pregnancy test from the first day of a missed period.

■ You may feel—or be—sick, not just in the morning. Your breasts may feel tender, you may need to urinate more often, you may be constipated, feel tired, or have a strange metallic taste in your mouth. You may go off tea, coffee, alcohol, or fatty foods.

■ See your doctor as soon as you think you are pregnant. Don't take any medication without taking his advice. If you are not yet taking folic acid supplements, start now. If you don't know whether you are immune to rubella, find out.

■ Drink plenty of water and make sure you have enough fiber in your diet to ward off constipation. Eat plenty of fresh fruit and vegetables and check the eating advice in Chapter Two to make sure you and your baby get all the nutrients you need. Don't fight tiredness—take catnaps if necessary and have early nights. By the end of week eight your baby is no longer known as an embryo, but a fetus. By now all his main internal organs are developing, he has a head and a trunk and a recognizable face. Dental buds are growing in each jaw.

8—12 WEEKS

■ During this time the placenta begins to function. Oxygen and food from your bloodstream pass into your baby's bloodstream via the umbilical cord. Antibodies, giving resistance to infection,

Opposite: the moment you have been waiting for. Pregnancy and birth are over and it is time for those first precious moments when you begin to bond.

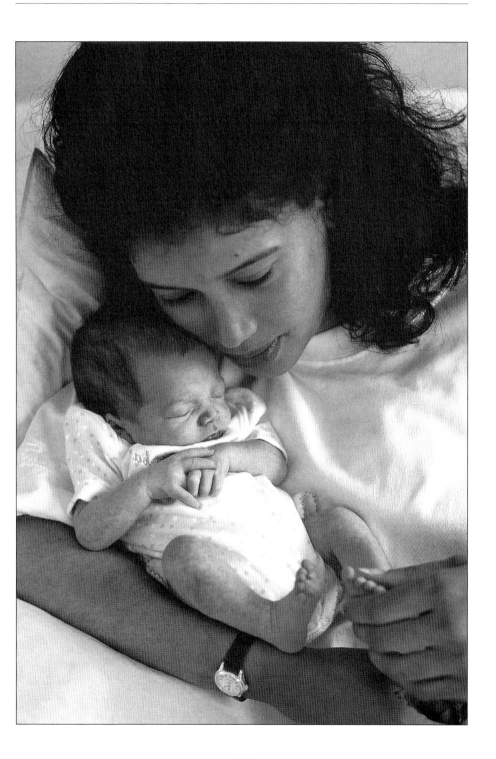

pass this way, too—but so can alcohol, nicotine, and other drugs.

■ By the end of the twelfth week the fetus is fully formed. From now on, he will grow rapidly.

■ The hormonal changes in your body may make your skin look smoother—but your gums may be getting softer too. Now is the time to start being particularly careful about dental hygiene. You may wish to make an appointment with your dentist.

■ You will probably attend your first antenatal appointment during this period and may be offered a number of different tests. You don't have to have any of these, although they are all done with the aim of making your pregnancy safer. You need to think about the kind of antenatal care you want, and where and how you'd like to have your baby.

■ If you want to try to reduce stretch marks, start to massage them with oil or cream now. Watch your diet, go on eating healthily, and make sure you are getting some exercise. If you are feeling sick, read the advice on page 52.

12—16 WEEKS

■ Your baby will now be growing rapidly. He is beginning to get hair as well as eyebrows and eyelashes.

■ If you have been feeling tired and sick you should start to feel better now. Your breasts will probably be getting bigger: get yourself a good supportive bra.

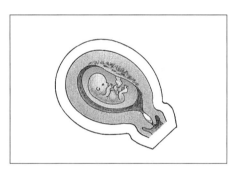

By the thirteenth week, your baby is four inches long, and attached to the placenta.

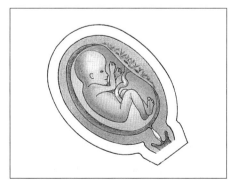

By the sixteenth week, your baby is growing fast and now has some hair.

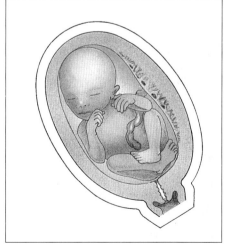

The twentieth week and your baby weighs 12 ounces and is ten inches long.

■ Find out about antenatal classes and make sure you are eating well and keeping fit. Make sure you have plenty of fiber in your diet to ward off constipation (see page 47).

■ You may feel warmer and sweatier than usual because of the hormonal changes and the increase in blood supply to your skin. Wear loose clothing made of natural fibers when you can.

■ Some pregnant women suffer from fainting. Try not to stand for too long and get up slowly when you are sitting or have been in a hot bath.

16—22 WEEKS

■ At some point after the sixteenth week you will feel the first butterfly movements as the baby will have started testing his reflexes, kicking, and stretching. Your uterus will now have grown so much that you will begin to look pregnant.

■ Make sure you are practicing your pelvic floor exercises (page 28). Foot exercises may help prevent cramp (page 48). Think about swimming or walking to keep fit and active.

22—28 WEEKS

■ You may feel hungrier than you used to. Don't abandon your balanced diet—eat fresh fruit and vegetables if you must snack. Your most rapid weight gain will take place during this time and your feet

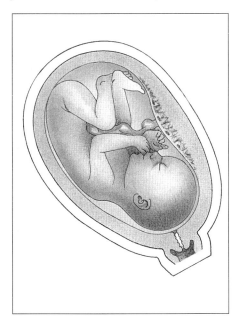

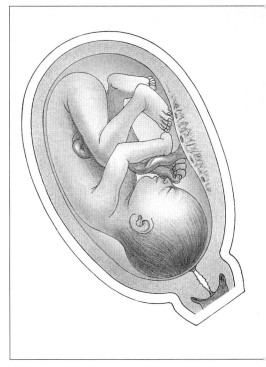

The twenty-fourth week and your baby looks much as he will at birth, albeit thinner.

By the thirty-second week, your baby is fatter and weighs about four pounds.

and legs may start to feel the strain. You may need shoes that are a size larger than normal. Do regular exercises to prevent varicose veins developing (page 54).

■ Your baby will start to move more vigorously now and will respond to touch and sound. He may be most active when you are resting, so you may find it difficult to get off to sleep at night. At twenty-four weeks your baby's vital organs are already well enough developed that he would have a chance of survival if he was born prematurely.

28—32 WEEKS

■ As your baby gets bigger you may find that you start to suffer from indigestion and heartburn (see page 49). Watch your posture when you are standing or sitting. See page 44 for tips on how to avoid and relieve backache.

■ Your womb may now be putting pressure on your bladder, making you feel the need to pass water often. Some women find it helpful to rock backward and forward when they are on the toilet, which lessens the pressure and helps empty the

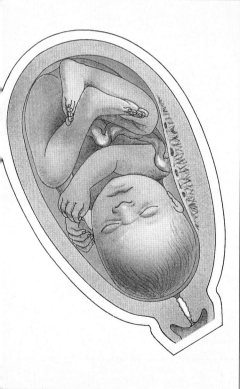

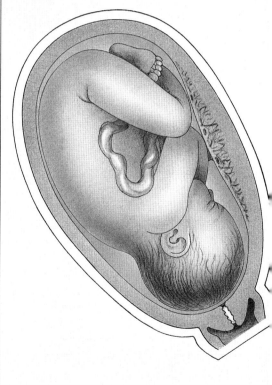

After week thirty-two your baby will turn round so he is head down.

By week thirty-six your baby is fully formed and is ready for birth.

bladder properly. Make sure you are still doing your pelvic floor exercises regularly to prevent stress incontinence. If you are going to go to antenatal classes, you should be starting them soon.

33—36 WEEKS
■ By now your baby is perfectly formed, but is still laying down his fat reserves beneath the skin.
■ This is the time to start practicing the relaxation and breathing exercises you plan to use in labor. You could also begin to experiment with positions you might want to adopt. When you can, rest

with your feet up to stop your ankles swelling (see page 51).

37—40 WEEKS
■ Once your baby's head engages you may find it easier to eat and breathe, but it may now feel uncomfortable to sit down. You may be getting strong practice contractions and the sheer effort of moving your increased weight about may make you feel very tired. Rest when you can and go to bed early. Massage and relaxation techniques may help you unwind and sleep. Make the most of these last days to build up your physical and emotional resources.

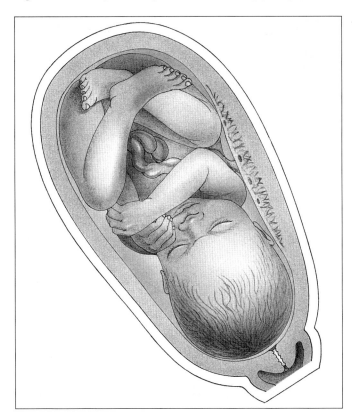

The moment has arrived at last and birth is imminent. Your baby will not move much because there is very little room. During the birth process, he will pass through the birth canal and into the outside world.

USEFUL ADDRESSES

UNITED STATES

ACUPUNCTURE
American Medical Acupuncture Association
7535 Laurel Canyon
Boulevard, Suite C
North Hollywood
CA 91605

CHIROPRACTIC
American Chiropractic Association
1701 Clarendon Boulevard
Arlington
VA 22209
Tel: (800) 986–4636

HERBAL THERAPY
The American Herbalists Guild
P.O. Box 1683
Soquel
CA 95073
Tel: (408) 464–2441

HOMEOPATHY
International Foundation for Homeopathy
2366 Eastlake Avenue
Suite 325
Seattle
WA 98102

Tel: (206) 324–8230

MASSAGE
American Massage Therapy Association
820 Davis Street
Suite 100
Evanston
IL 60201–4444
Tel: (708) 864–0123

OSTEOPATHY
American Osteopathic Association
142 E Ontario Street
Chicago
IL 60611

REFLEXOLOGY
International Institute of Reflexology
P.O. Box 12642
St. Petersburg
FL 33733–2642
Tel: (813) 343–4811

UNITED KINGDOM

COMPLEMENTARY MEDICINE
The Institute for Complementary Medicine

P.O. Box 194
London SE16 1QZ
Tel: 0171 237 5165
Send a stamped addressed envelope and two loose stamps to the Information Office if you need to find out about complementary practitioners and courses.

For information on registered practitioners in most forms of Complementary Medicine, you should contact:
The British Register of Complementary Practitioners
P.O. Box 194
London SE16 1QZ

ALEXANDER TECHNIQUE
Society of Teachers of the Alexander Technique
20 London House
Fulham Road
London SW10 9EL
Tel: 0171 351 0828

AUTOGENIC TRAINING
For details of local trainers write to:
British Association for

Autogenic Training and Therapy (BAFATT)
18 Holtsmere Close
Garston
Watford
Herts WD2 6NG

CHIROPRACTIC
British Chiropractic Association
29 Whitley Street
Reading
Berkshire
RG2 0EG
Tel: 01734 757557

HERBALISM
The National Institute of Medical Herbalists
9 Palace Gate
Exeter
Devon
EX1 1JA
Tel: 01392 426022

NATUROPATHY
The General Council and Register of Naturopaths
Goswell House
2 Goswell Road
Street
Somerset BA16 0JG
Tel: 01458 840072

OSTEOPATHY
General Council and Register of Osteopaths

56 London Street
Reading
Berkshire RG1 4SQ
Tel: 01734 576585

PHYSIOTHERAPY
The Association of Chartered Physiotherapists in Obstetrics and Gynaecology
14 Bedford Row
London
WC1R 4ED
Tel: 0171 242 1941

PhysioFirst (the organisation of chartered physiotherapists in private practice)
8 Weston Chambers
Weston Road
Southend-on-Sea
Essex SS1 1AT
Tel: 01702 392124

YOGA
The Iyengar Yoga Institute
223a Randolph Avenue
London W9 1NL
Tel: 0171 624 3080

OTHER USEFUL INFORMATION

PRECONCEPTION
For information and advice on

preconceptual care, contact:
Foresight
28 The Paddock
Godalming
Surrey GU7 1XD
Tel: 01483 427839

SMOKING
For help to stop smoking, read the free Health Education Authority booklet *Stopping Smoking Made Easier.* Or for details of local support services, phone **Quitline** on:
England: 0800 002200
Scotland: 0800 84 84 84
Wales: 0345 697 500

ASH (Action on Smoking and Health)
109 Gloucester Place
London
W1H 3PH
Tel: 0171 935 3519

GENERAL
Toxoplasmosis Trust
61 Collier Street, London
N1 9BE
Helpline: 0171 713 0599

Employment Medical Advisory Service: confidential advice about reproductive hazards at work. Run by Health and

Safety Executive. Check phone book for local HQ.

National Childbirth Trust
Alexandra House
Oldham Terrace
London W3 6NH
Tel: 0181 992 8637
Runs antenatal classes giving information about labor, relaxation, massage and active positions for birth. Also publishes range of useful booklets. Local branches.

Association for Improvements in the Maternity Services (AIMS)
Support and information about rights and choices.
England and Wales:
40 Kingswood Avenue
London NW6 6LS
Tel: 0181 960 5585

Scotland:
40 Leamington Terrace
Edinburgh EH10 4JL
Tel: 0131 229 6259
Eire:
18 Firgrove Drive
Bishopstown
Cork
Tel: 00353 21342649
Northern Ireland:
23 Station Mews
Todd's Hill
Saintfield
Co Down
Tel: 01238 511786

Active Birth Centre
25 Bickerton Road
London N19 5JT
Tel: 0171 561 9006
Runs pregnancy yoga classes, courses on preparing for labor and birth, active birth and water birth workshops. Also has a nationwide pool hire

service, a register of certified active birth teachers, and a range of books, aromatherapy, and herbal products which can be bought by mail order.

The Nutri Centre
7 Park Crescent
London W1N 3HE
Tel: 0171 436 5122
Mail order catalogue for all alternative and complementary health products.

Maternity Alliance
45 Beech Street
London EC2P 2LX
Tel: 0171 588 8582
Information leaflets include Good Beginnings, a healthy food guide in pregnancy, Getting Fit for Pregnancy and Health and Safety at Work, your rights in pregnancy and after childbirth.

FURTHER READING/VIDEOS

Enjoy Healthy Eating, Health Education Authority, free from doctors or clinics.
Every Woman's Birth Rights, Pat Thomas (Thorsons).
The Postnatal Exercise Book, Margie Polden and Barbara Whiteford, (Frances Lincoln).
BBC Pregnancy and Postnatal Exercise Video, written and produced by obstetric

physiotherapists.
Your Baby, Your Choice—a guide to planning your labor, available from the Maternity Alliance (see above).
Choices in Childbirth Pack. Includes information about rights and choices as well as booklets on choosing a home birth or a water birth. Available from AIMS (see above).

INDEX

A

Acupressure, 51, 52, 95

Acupuncture, 8, 51, 52, 87, 95

Additives, 10

Alcohol, 8, 10, 102

Alexander Technique, 95

Allergy, 20

Anaemia, 20

Ankles, swollen, 100

Antenatal classes, 58, 105

Antibodies, 102

Anxiety, 100

Arnica, 48, 92

Aromatherapy, 12, 47, 51, 54, 95–96

massage, 12, 49,

Autogenic Training, 96

B

Bach Flower Remedies, 96–97

Bach Rescue Remedy, 87

Backache, 44, 67, 95, 96, 100

Birth, natural, 70

Bladder, 107

Breasts, caring for, 66

Breathing, 70

controled, 100

exercises, 50, 107

in labor, 86

techniques, 60–66

transitional, 66

Breathlessness, 47

Breech babies, 95

Bridging, 41

C

Caesarean, 78, 80, 84

Caffeine, 10, 22

Calcium, 11, 20

Candida, 6

Carbohydrates, 19

Carbon disulphide, 14

Carbon monoxide, 14, 22

Cereals, whole-grain, 19

Cervical smear, 6

Chemicals, 14

Chiropractic, 47, 97

Cocaine, 8

Coffee, 10, 22

Cola, 10, 22

Colostrum, 66

Color therapy, 97

Colorings, 10

Computer terminals, 14

Conception, 102

Constipation, 47, 98, 100

Contraception, 6, 8, 14

Contractions,

breathing for, 65

Copper, 14

Counseling, 8

Cramp, 48, 98

Cranial osteopathy, 78, 98

Cravings, 18

Cycling, 25, 54

D

Dental work, 15, 54

Diet, 10–11, 16–23, 56

Drinking habits, 8

Drugs, 8, 22

E

Ecstasy, 8

Electronic monitoring, 81

Environmental hazards, 14–15, 102

Epidural, 83–84

Episiotomy, 66, 91

Essential oils, 12–13, 49, 95–96

Exercise(s), 24–43, 47, 51

pelvic floor, 28

strengthening, 37–43

F

Fainting, 105

Fatigue, 49, 96, 98, 100

Fats, 22

Fertility, 8, 10

Fiber, 19, 47

Fluid retention, 51, 95

Folic acid, 10, 20, 102

Forceps delivery, 80, 84

Formaldehyde, 14

G

Gas and air, 82

German measles, 6, 102

H

Hemorrhoids, 51

Hair, 52–53

Health checks, preconceptual, 6, 102

Heart disease, 22

Heartbeat, monitoring baby's, 80–81

Heartburn, 49–50, 98

Herbal medicine, 8, 47, 51, 52, 54, 87, 91, 98

Herbal teas, 48

HIV virus, 6

Home births, 91

Homeopathy, 6–8, 47, 48, 50, 51, 52, 54, 78, 87, 98

Hormonal changes, 52

Hospital birth, 72–91

Hypnotherapy, 8

I

Indigestion, 49–50

Insecticides, 14

Insomnia, 50, 96, 97, 98, 100

Iron, 20

Iyenga yoga, 100

K

Kali Carbonica, 47

L
Labor, 24, 25, 44,
56, 78, 80–91
breathing for, 62–66
choices in, 78
pain relief in, 82–87
positions for, 67–69,
70, 77, 88–90
relaxation in, 86–87
speeding up, 78
stages of, 78
Laxatives, 47
Lead, 14
Lifting, 45
Listeria, 21

M
Magnesium, 11
Marijuana, 8
Massage, 47, 51, 87
aromatherapy, 12
Meditation, 12
Mercury, 15
Metals, toxic, 14
Milk, 10,
allergy, 20
Minerals, 10–11
Miscarriage, 8, 14, 25
Missed period, 102

N
Natural birth, 70
Naturopathy, 51, 98
Nausea, 52, 96
Neural tube defects,
19
Nicotine, 22
Nose bleeds, 50–51

Nubane, 82

O
Oedema, 51, 98
Osteopathy, 47, 100

P
Pain relief, 82–87
Pelvic floor exercises,
28, 107
Pelvic rocking, 46
Perineum massage, 66
Period problems, 14
Pesticides, 14, 19
Pethidine, 84
Pharmaceuticals, 14
Piles, 51, 98
Placenta, 90, 91
Positions for labor,
66–69, 70, 77,
88–90
Posture, 45, 46, 100
Preconception, 102
Preconceptual care,
6–15
Pregnancy sickness,
52
Premature babies, 22
Preparing for
pregnancy, 6–15

R
Radiation screens, 14
Rectal separation,
testing for, 37
Reflexology, 8, 47, 100
Relaxation, 8, 12,
29–31, 50, 56,

100, 102
in labor, 61, 70,
86–87
touch, 60–61
Rubella, 6, 102

S
Sea-Bands, 52
Sexual dysfunction,
14
Sexually transmitted
diseases, 6
Skin, 52–53
complaints, 98
Sleeping, 56–57, 100
Smoking, 8, 14, 22
passive, 15
Sperm counts, 8
Sperm damage, 14
Starchy food, 19
Sterility, 14
Stillbirths, 14
Stress, 8, 12–13, 24,
100, 102
Stretch marks, 53,
104
Sugar, 10, 22
Support bra, 104
Swimming, 25, 54
Swollen ankles, 100
Syntometrine, 91

T
Tea, 10
Teeth and gums, 54
Tennis, 25
Testosterone, 8
Thrush, 6, 54

Tiredness, 8
Touch relaxation,
60–61
Toxoplasmosis, 21
Transitional breathing,
66

U
Ultrasound detectors,
81

V
Varicose veins, 54, 98,
106
Visualization, 86–87
Vitamins, 10, 11, 18,
19, 20, 21
supplements, 10,
20–21

W
Walking, 54
Water, 10
births, 91
filters, 10
Weight, 10–11
gain in pregnancy,
17, 105
Workplace, 15

X
X-rays, 15

Y
Yoga, 8, 100

Z
Zinc, 10, 14